CW0051711?

AUTHOR'S ADDRESS

It is with deep sense of gratitude, humility, and fulfillment that I present this book to you, esteemed reader.

This book, Comprehensive Handbook of Bacteriology, is loaded with essential, high yield and clinically optimized information about all Bacteria of Medical Importance. Kindly see our table of contents for details.

The book is a complex extract from standard texts of Medical Bacteriology. It is carefully written in a friendly, easily comprehensible and logically sequential manner, using tables and illustrations that enhance easy understanding.

I promise you will really enjoy studying Bacteriology using this book. If you did enjoy it, I will be very grateful if you would post a short review on Amazon. Thank you!!!

With Gratitude,
Karen Morse.

TABLE OF CONTENTS

CHAPTER 1: INTRODUCTION TO BACTERIOLOGY

❖ BACTERIAL TAXONOMY

− Taxonomy is a science that deals with the classification, nomenclature and identification of microorganisms
− Bacteria are the most widely studied groups of microorganisms; thus their taxonomy is the most advanced
− It is pertinent to explain further the contextual meaning of the following:

▪ Classification

− This refers to orderly arrangement of organisms into taxonomic groups, based on their similarities
− Taxonomic groups are: kingdom, phylum, class, order, family, genus, species

▪ Nomenclature

− This is the naming of an organism based on its characteristics, as genus and specie, using international rules

▪ Identification

− This refers to the practical use of a classification scheme to isolate and distinguish organisms, verify the authenticity of a culture or isolate and identify the causative agent of a disease

● Definition of terms

Term	Definition
Specie	A group of organisms that closely resemble one another in the more important features of their organisation
Strain	A line of genetically different bacteria presumed to descend from a single ancestral bacterium
Clone	A pure culture considered to consist exclusively of the progeny of a single cell and does not include any demonstrable mutant cell i.e. are genetically identical

Isolate	A primary culture of an organism from its natural source e.g. soil

- **Nomenclature in bacteriology**
- Naming of bacterial specie is done in accordance with the principles and rules of nomenclature set forth in the Bacteriological Code
- The scientific name must be in Greek or Latin word
- The genus name begins with a capital letter and the specie name with a small letter
- The names should either be italicized or underlined, but not both
- For example: *Staphylococcus aureus* or Staphylococcus aureus

❖ **MORPHOLOGY OF BACTERIA**
- Generally, bacteria cells occur in four major shapes; which may organizes themselves to give more complex structures (see fig 1.1)

▪ **Cocci**
- Spherical bacteria
- They may appear singly, or associate in pairs, chains or clusters i.e. diplococcus, streptococcus and staphylococcus respectively
- For instance, *Neisseria meningitis, Streptococcus Pneumonia* and *Staphylococcus aureus* occur in pairs, chains and clusters respectively

▪ **Bacilli**
- Rod-shaped bacteria
- They may appear singly or associate in chains
- For instance, *Bacillus anthracis* and members of the genus streptobacillus typically occur in chains

- Coccobacilli are very short rod-shaped bacteria, that may be mistaken for cocci (fig 1.1)

- Vibrio
- Comma (curved-rod) shaped bacteria
- Examples are *Vibrio cholerae*, *Vibrio parahaemolyticus* etc.

- Spirillum/spirochete
- Spiral-shaped bacteria
- Called spirilla if cells are rigid e.g. *Spirillum minus*
- Called spirochetes if cells are more flexible and undulating e.g. *Treponema pallidum*

❖ GRAM STAIN
- Gram staining is a differential staining procedure described in 1884 by Hans Christian Gram
- It forms the basis upon which bacteria are classified as gram-positive or gram-negative

- Gram staining mechanism
- Make a smear of the specimen onto a glass slide; then heat it to fix the bacteria
- Apply crystal violet stain (a purple dye) to the heat-fixed smear, and rinse off after 1 min (under a running tap)
- Add iodine solution to the smear and rinse it off after 1 min
- Decolorize the smear with alcohol or acetone and rinse off immediately
- Finally, counter-stain the smear with safranin (a red dye) and rinse off after 30 seconds

- Interpretation of results
- This is done by studying the smear under the microscope

- Gram-positive bacteria absorb and retain the crystal violet stain; thus appear purple
- Gram-negative bacteria does not retain the crystal violet stain, but absorb the safranin stain; thus appear red

✓ Note: iodine is serving as a mordant in Gram staining
✓ Mordant is a substance capable of combining with a stain to intensify the binding of the stain to the specimen

CHAPTER 2: NUMERICAL CLASSIFICATION OF BACTERIA

- **Classification of Bacteria (four main classes)**
- − True bacteria
- − False (filamentous) bacteria
- − Atypical bacteria
- − Miscellaneous bacteria

- ❖ **TRUE BACTERIA**
- − This is a large group bacteria characterised by possession of rigid cell walls
- − Based on morphology, they are divided into cocci and bacilli
- − Based on Gram staining, they are divided into gram-positive and gram-negative
- − Thus we have four subdivisions of true bacteria:
- - Gram-positive cocci
- - Gram-negative cocci
- - Gram-positive bacilli
- - Gram-negative bacilli

- **Gram-positive cocci**

- **Examples include:**
- − Staphylococcus − *S. aureus, S. epidermidis, S. saprophyticus* etc.
- − Streptococcus − *S. agalactiae, S. bovis, S. canis, S. pneumoniae, S. pyogenes* etc.
- − Micrococcus
- − Peptococcus
- − Peptostreptococcus

- **Gram-negative cocci**

- Examples include:
  - Neisseria – *N. gonorrhoeae, N. meningitidis* etc.
  - Moraxella – *M. catarrhalis* etc.
  - Veillonella – *V. parvula* etc.

- **Gram-positive bacilli**
  - Based on their oxygen requirement for metabolism, members of this group are divided into aerobes and anaerobes
  - Each of them is further divided into spore-forming and nonspore-forming bacteria
  - Thus we have four subdivisions of gram-positive bacilli:

- Aerobic spore-forming gram-positive bacilli
  - Bacillus - *B cereus, B. anthracis* etc.

- Aerobic nonspore-forming gram-positive bacilli
  - Corynebacterium – *C. diphtheriae, C. jeikeium* etc.
  - Listeria – *L. monocytogenes* etc.
  - Erysipelothrix

- Anaerobic spore-forming gram-positive bacilli
  - Clostridium – *C. tetani, C. botulinum, C. difficile* etc.

- Anaerobic nonspore-forming gram-positive bacilli
  - Lactobacillus
  - Leptotrichia
  - Propionibacterium – *P. acnes* etc.
  - Bifidobacterium

- **Gram-negative bacilli**
  - As for the Gram-positive bacilli, members of this group are divided into aerobes and anaerobes

- Thus we have two subdivisions of gram-negative bacilli:

• Aerobic gram-negative bacilli
- Pseudomonas – *P. aeruginosa, P. fluorescens* etc.
- Burkholderia.

• Anaerobic gram-negative bacilli
- This group is further divided into two:

✓ **Strictly anaerobic gram-negative bacilli**
- Bacteroides – *B. fragilis* etc.
- Prevotella – *P. melaninogenica* etc.
- Porphyromonas – *P. gingivalis* etc.

✓ **Facultative   anaerobic   gram-negative   bacilli (enterobacteriaceae)**
- Escherichia
- Klebsiella
- Salmonella
- Shigella
- Enterobacter
- Morganella
- Serratia

❖ FILAMENTOUS BACTERIA
- Examples include:
• Actinomyces
• Streptomyces

❖ ATYPICAL BACTERIA
- Examples include:
- Mycoplasma
- Ureaplasma

- Chlamydia
- Rickettsia

❖ **MISCELLANEOUS BACTERIA**
- These are sub-classified into five groups

Group	Examples
Gram-negative	Afipia Bartonella Streptobacillus Gardnerella Calymmatobacterium
Gram-negative coccobacilli	Haemophilus – *H. influenza* Bordetella – *B. pertussis* Brucella – *B. abortus, B. canis, B. melitensis* etc
Acid-fast bacilli	Mycobacteria – *M. tuberculosis, M. leprae, M. bovis* etc. Nocardia
Curved rods	Vibrio – *V. cholerae* Campylobacter Helicobacter Arcobacter
Spiral-shaped	Spirilla – *S. minus* Spirochaetes- Borrelia, Treponema, Leptospira

T

CHAPTER 3: STRUCTURE AND FUNCTION OF BACTERIA CELL

- ▪ Introduction
- – Bacteria are microorganisms with prokaryotic form of cellular organisation; seen only with the aid of microscope
- – Generally, they are unicellular organisms but they grow attached to one another in clusters, chains, rods or filaments.
- – They possess a relatively rigid cell wall that maintains their characteristic shape as coccus, bacillus, vibrio or spirillum and spirochete

- ▪ Characteristics of bacteria cell

- ● Rigid cell wall
- – Made of peptidoglycan a.k.a. murein, mucopeptide etc.

- ● Simple nucleus (nucleoid)
- – Has no membrane
- – Lacks nucleolus and mitotic spindle; thus incapable of mitosis
- – Division is by binary fission

- ● Absent internal membranes
- – Cytoplasmic structures are not demarcated from one another
- – This accounts for their ability to carry out both transcription and translation simultaneously

- ❖ ULTRA-STRUCTURE OF BACTERIA
  - – This can be appreciated only under electron microscope (EM)
- – The bacterial cell consist of two major parts:
- ● Protoplasm
- ● Nuclear material

▪ **Nuclear Material**

● **Bacterial chromosome**

– Single, supercoiled, circular double-stranded DNA found in bacteria nucleoid
– Being single makes it is an haploid; about 1000μm in length
– It is not membrane-bound, but attaches to invaginations of the cytoplasmic membrane
– It lacks histone protein and thus, does not stain
– It stores genetic information for bacterial structure, functions and replication
– It is able to express changes, and get rid of mutations easily

● **Extra-chromosomal genetic material**

– These are genetic material within the bacterial cytoplasm
– They include:

● **Plasmids**

– They are circular double-stranded DNA molecules
– They are autonomous i.e. can replicate independent of bacterial chromosome
– They code for antibiotic and heavy metal resistance, conjugation, toxin production etc.
– However, they are not essential for cell vitality

● **Transposons (a.k.a. jumping genes)**

– They are linear double-stranded DNA molecule
– They depend on bacterial chromosome or plasmid for their replication
– Like plasmid, they code for special bacterial characters

- Episomes
- These are plasmids that can behave like transposons i.e. can detach and attach to bacterial chromosomes, and yet have self-replicating ability

- Protoplasm
- A body of living material made up of **cytoplasm**
- It is surrounded by **cell envelope**
- It may give rise to **cell appendages** (flagella or pili)

- Cytoplasm
- A viscous watery solution, containing variety of solutes, and numerous granules called ribosomes
- Unlike in eukaryotes, it lacks organelles e.g. mitochondria, Golgi body etc.
- It shows no sign of internal mobility, seen in eukaryotes

✓ **Ribosomes**
- They are seen as small granules in the cytoplasm; 10 – 20nm in size
- They are strunged together on strands of mRNA as polysomes
- Each of the ribosome within a polysome is called monosome
- Each bacteria ribosome consist of two subunits; a large subunit (50S) and a small subunit (30S) both of which sediment at 70S
- "S" is Svedberg unit; each unit equals to 10^{-13} second
- Aminoglycosides inhibit the 30S subunit, while macrolides inhibit the 50S subunit

✓ **Cytoplasmic inclusion bodies**
- These are aggregates of excess metabolites, stored within the cytoplasm as nutrient reserves
- They are not found in all bacteria, and not everytime in the same bacteria

- Their presence depends on accessibility to energy yielding nutrient
- Examples of such metabolite include:
- Volutin granule a.k.a. metachromatic granules – composed of polyphosphates
- Lipid granules –composed of poly β-hydroxyl butyric acid
- Polysaccharide granules – composed of glycogen or starch

- Cell Envelope
- Bacterial cell envelope comprise cytoplasmic membrane, cell wall and or capsule

- Cytoplasmic membrane
- An elastic structure, about 5 – 10nm in thickness, limiting the protoplasm externally
- Made of lipoprotein; arranged as phospholipid bilayer with inner and outer protein layers
- Thus, it appears under EM as two electron-dense layer (protein) separated by an electroluscent layer (lipid)
- It is similar to eukaryote cell membrane; only that it lacks sterol
- Exception is Mycoplasma which can incorporate sterol upon itself

- Function
- As an osmotic barrier: it maintains differences between solute contents of the cytoplasm and the exterior
- As a permeability barrier: it allow passive diffusion of lipid soluble substances and selective active transport of specific nutrients and waste product in and out of the cell
- Acts as storage site for biosynthetic enzymes, cytochrome enzymes, transport proteins etc.

■ Mesosomes
- These are convoluted membranous bodies
- Formed by invaginations of the cytoplasmic membrane into the cytoplasm
- They are divided into two: septal and Lateral mesosomes
- They are designed to compartmentalize the DNA during cell division (septal mesosome), provide support for respiratory enzymes and to remove waste products from the cytoplasm

❖ Cell wall
- This rigid structure lies immediately outside the cytoplasmic membrane
- Measures about 10 – 25nm in thickness and allows passage of solutes < 1nm in thickness

■ Function
- Protects the cell membrane against the high osmotic pressure of the protoplasm (5 – 20 atm)
- Maintains the characteristic shape of the bacteria
- It plays an essential role in essential in cell division

■ Structure of cell wall
- The structure of bacterial cell is can be conveniently divided into two:
• Basal structure (peptidoglycan)
• Specialized structure

• Basal structure (peptidoglycan)
- This is a complex of peptide and glycan
- It has three structural parts:

✓ **Glycan (straight) chain**
- The back bone of the structure

- Made of repeating units of N-acetyl glucosamine and N-acetyl muramic acid
- It is the same in all bacterial species

✓ **Tetraptide (side) chains**

- A set of identical tetrapeptide; they vary from species to species
- They attach to N-acetyl muramic acid portion of the glycan chain
- In most gram-positive bacteria it is composed of: L-alanine, D-glutamate, L-lysine, D-alanine
- For gram-negative bacteria, diaminopimelic acid replaces L-lysine at position 3

✓ **Cross bridges**

- A set of identical peptides that attaches one straight chain to the other via the side chain
- it vary from species to species
- in *Staphylococcus aureus*, it is a pentaglycine bond

• **Specialized structures**

- These are a.k.a. supporting structures
- They are best described separately for gram-positive and gram-negative bacteria

✓ **Specialized structures of gram-positive bacteria**

- Teichoic acid – polymers of glycerol or ribitol phosphate
- Teichuronic acid – a techoic acid-like polymer that lacks phosphate group
- Polysaccharides

✓ **Specialized structures of gram-negative bacteria**

- Outer membrane

- Lipopolysaccharide (LPS)
- Lipoprotein
- Periplasmic space

* **Outer membrane of gram-negative bacteria**
- It is a bilayered structure; its inner leaflet has compositions similar to normal cell membrane
- The outer leaflet contains a distinctive component called lipopolysaccharide (LPS)

* **Lipopolysaccharide (LPS)**
- Lipopolysaccharide a.k.a. endotoxin, is made of two parts: Lipid A and polysaccharide
- Lipid A is the toxic fatty acid part; it solely account for the endotoxic shock associated with these organisms
- Polysaccharide part a.k.a. O antigen is highly immunogenic; it induces antibodies formation

* **Periplasmic space**
- This is the space between the inner and outer membrane
- It contains the peptidoglycan layer, β-lactamase, binding proteins, iron, vitamin B_{12} etc.

■ **Difference between gram-positive and gram-negative cell wall**

Characteristics	Gram-positive cell wall	Gram-negative cell wall
Thickness	Thick	Thin
Number of layers	One	Two
Peptidoglycan	30-40 sheet	2-3 sheets

Outer membrane	Absent	Present
Periplasmic space	Absent	Present
Techoic acid	Present	Absent
Protein	Absent	Present
Lipid	Less	More
Toxins produced	Primarily exotoxin	Primarily endotoxin
Susceptibility to antimicrobial agents	High	Low
Gram staining	Purple	Red

- **Cell wall deficient bacteria**
- These are a.k.a. L-form bacteria
- They are formed when bacteria are treated with enzymes e.g. lysozyme or antibiotics e.g. penicillin that are lytic to the cell wall; though, others form spontaneously
- There are two types: stable L-form and unstable L-form

- Stable L-form
- Once they form, they do not revert back to the parent cell
- Example is *Streptobacillus moniliformis*; the causative agent of rat-bite fever

- Unstable L-form
- They can revert back to the parent cell
- Examples are protoplasts (from gram-positive bacteria) and spheroplasts (from gram-negative bacteria)
- mycoplasmas

- **CAPSULE**
- This firm gelatinous material lie outside and immediately in contact with the cell envelope

- It is a polysaccharide except in *Bacillus anthracis* where it is made of poly D-glutamic acid
- It protects the cell wall against antibiotics, and the bacteria against ingestion by phagocytes
- It is immunogenic; as it bears the K-antigen

- **CELL APPENDAGES**
- These are the flagella and pili

- Flagella
- Flagella is made of protein subunits called flagellin
- It originate from the protoplasm and extruded through the cell wall
- It is highly antigenic; as it bears the H-antigen
- It serves as organ of locomotion for the bacteria that possess them
- Depending on the bacterial specie, it is may be between 1 – 20 per cell

✓ **Types of flagella arrangement**
- Monotrichous – single polar flagellum e.g. *Vibrio cholerae*
- Lopotrichous - multiple polar flagella e.g. *Helicobacter pylori*
- Peritrichous –flagella distributed over the entire cell e.g. *Proteus vulgaris*

- Pili (Fimbriae)
- Pili is made of protein subunits called pilins
- They are shorter, finer and more numerous (100 -500 per cell) than the flagella
- It is possessed by many gram-negative bacteria e.g. *Neisseria gonorrhoeae*

- They serve as organ of adhesion
- A specialized pili (sex pilus) serves as organ of conjugation

CHAPTER 4: INTRODUCTION TO BACTERIAL GENETICS

- Genetics is the study of inheritance and variation
- Bacterial genetics is a subfield of genetics, devoted to study of hereditary mechanisms in bacteria
- It forms the basis for modern genetic engineering and molecular biology

- Genetic variations in bacteria
- Genetic variations in bacteria occur as a result of two main mechanisms:
  - Mutation
  - Gene transfer

❖ MUTATION
- Though the DNA is believed to be a stable structure, some occasional inaccuracies in replication may occur, producing a slight alteration in the nucleotide sequence of one of the daughter cells
- This inheritable change or alteration in the nucleotide sequence is termed mutation and the agent inducing it is called a mutagen

- Causes of mutation
- Spontaneous: - mutation which occurs naturally; it occurs in about one in every 10^6 to one in every 10^9 divisions
- Chemical mutagens: - e.g. 5-bromouracil, 2-aminouracil etc.
- Physical mutagen: - e.g. X-ray, ultraviolet light etc.
- Molecular biological techniques: - e.g. transposons, bacteriophage etc.

- **Types of mutation**

- **Point mutation**
  - This is the commonest type of mutation; in which a single base at one point in the DNA sequence is replaced by another base (i.e. base substitution)

- **Missense mutation**
  - This is a base substitution which results in an amino acid substitution in the synthesised protein;
  - Example is in the sickle β-globin gene; where adenine is substituted by thymine (base substitution) which result in substitution of glutamate by valine (amino acid substitution) in the synthesised hemoglobin

- **Non-sense mutation**
  - This is a base substitution which results in formation of stop codon; causing premature termination of protein synthesis
  - Only a fragment of the complete protein is formed; hence the term "non-sense"

- **Frame-shift mutation**
  - This is the insertion or deletion of one or few base pairs in the DNA sequence; causing a shift in the translational reading frame (codon)
  - This results in the synthesis of a long stretch of altered amino acids and in turn production of inactive protein

- ❖ **GENE TRANSFER IN BACTERIA**
  - A change in the genome of bacteria may be due either to a mutation in the organism's own DNA or acquisition of the DNA from an external source

- ▪ Mechanisms of gene transfer in bacteria
- – Bacteria DNA be it chromosome, plasmid or transposon may be transferred between species of bacteria by 3 main mechanisms:
  - Transformation
  - Transduction
  - Conjugation

- • Transformation
- – DNA may be released from a bacteria (either artificially or by lysis) into the environment; this is called naked DNA
- – Another bacterium of the same or different specie may incorporate a fragment of this naked DNA onto its own chromosome through the cell wall
- – This uptake of free or naked DNA from one bacterium directly into another bacterium is called transformation
- – It usually occur in the late logarithm growth phase of the bacteria
- – There are two types of transformation: natural and artificial
- – Natural transformation occurs in *Streptococcus pneumoniae, Haemophilus influenza, Neisseria gonorrhoeae, Bacillus spp.* etc.
- – Artificial is done in the laboratory

- • Transduction
- – This the transfer of gene from a donor bacterial cell to a recipient bacteria cell by a bacteriophage
- – Bacteriophages are viruses that parasitize and multiply in bacteria
- – There are two types of transduction: generalized and specialized (restricted)

- Generalized transduction can be seen in *Shigella spp., salmonella spp., E. coli, Pseudomonas spp., Staphylococcus spp., Bacillus spp.* etc.
- Restricted transduction can be seen in *E. coli*

- • Conjugation
- Here, a bacteria cell called donor or male makes contact with another called recipient or female to transfer the DNA directly through a specialized fimbrae called sex pilus
- The ability of a bacterium to act as a donor is determined by its possession of a transmissible plasmid a.k.a. sex or transfer factor
- The transmissible plasmid is first replicated within the male and a copy is transferred to the female via the sex pilus
- Thus, following conjugation, the recipient becomes a male and the donor remain a male
- *Neisseria gonorrhoeae* is the best example for this mechanism

CHAPTER 5: BACTERIAL GROWTH

- **Introduction**
  - Bacterial growth is the balanced increase in all the cellular constituents of a bacterium, leading to an increase in length and size of the cell
  - Division of the bacterium occurs when growth reaches a critical point
  - Thus bacteria growth is also referred to as an increase in size of the bacteria population and not mere increase in size of individual bacterium
  - Death of bacterial is due to the irreversible loss of ability to reproduce

- **Bacterial Division**
  - Bacteria divide by binary fission (fig 1.1)
  - When the bacteria grows to about twice its size, its chromosome duplicates
  - An invagination from the cell membrane (septal mesosome) then divides the cell into two
  - The daughter cells receive identical set of chromosomes, and rearrange singly, in pairs or chains etc.

- **Bacterial growth curve**
  - In other to study bacterial growth, they are cultivated in a batch culture
  - Batch culture is a closed culture system with specific nutrient, temperature, aeration and other environmental conditions to optimise growth.
  - Because nutrients are not added, nor waste products removed during the incubation, batch cultures can only complete limited number of life cycles before bacteria die out

- The logarithm of the number of viable cells in the batch culture can be plotted against the time of incubation (during which count is made) on the bacterial growth curve (fig 5.1)
- The resulting curve has four distinct phases:
  - Lag phase
  - Log/exponential phase
  - stationary phase
  - Death /decline phase

- **Lag phase**
- In this phase, there is increase in cell size but no multiplication
- The organisms are trying to adapt to their new environment
- Enzymes, ribosomes, and other essential molecules are synthesised and accumulate until they are enough to permit division
- Antibiotics have little effect here

- **Log/exponential phase**
- In this phase, the cells grow and multiply at the maximum rate possible
- Multiplication occurs in geometric progression i.e. 2^0, 2^1, 2^2, 2^3..... 2^n; where n is the number of generation
- Generation time a.k.a. doubling time is the average time required for the population to double
- Growth in this phase is referred to as balanced growth; as cellular constituents are synthesised at a relatively constant rate
- However, if nutrient level decrease or other environmental changes occur, unbalanced growth results
- Antibiotics work better at this phase

- **Stationary phase**
- This phase is characterised by balance between growth rate and death rate

- It occurs due either to severe depletion of essential nutrients or accumulation of toxic metabolites in the medium
- It is important to know that, production of exotoxins, antibiotics, spores and metachromatic granules occur in this phase

- **Death or decline phase**
- In this phase, there is progressive death of cells
- The number of viable cells decreases geometrically (i.e. at exponential rate), like the reverse of growth in the log phase
- It was assumed that the cells suffered an irreparable damage, and if they were transferred to fresh medium, no cellular growth was noticed

CHAPTER 6: ANTIMICROBIAL CHEMOTHERAPY

▪ **Introduction**
- Antimicrobial agent is any substance capable of killing or inhibiting the growth of microorganisms
- Antimicrobial chemotherapy is the treatment of infections with antimicrobial agent specific for the infecting pathogen

▪ **Properties of an ideal antimicrobial agent**
- Selective toxicity – most important
- Should be soluble in body fluids
- Must not be inactivated by gastric acid
- Must not have significant effect on resident microflora of the host
- Should not be easy to develop resistance against

• **Selective toxicity**
- This means the drug should be effective against the target pathogen without having any harmful effect on the host

▪ **Classification of antimicrobial agent**
- Antimicrobial agents are classified into four, based on the microorganism they primarily affect:
  • Antibacterial agents / Antibiotics
  • Antifungal agents
  • Antiviral agents
  • Antiparasitic agents

❖ **ANTIBACTERIAL AGENTS / ANTIBIOTICS**
- Antibacterial agents are naturally occurring or semi-synthetic chemical substances capable, in dilute solution, of killing or inhibiting the growth of bacteria

- ■ Classification of antibiotics
- − Antibiotics may be classified on any of the following basis:
- • Mechanism of action
- • Spectrum of activity − broad / narrow / limited spectrum
- • Whether they kill or inhibit the organism − bacteriocidal / bacteriostatic

- • Classification based on mechanism of action
- − Inhibitors of cell wall synthesis
- − Inhibitors of cell membrane function
- − Inhibitors of protein synthesis
- − Inhibitors of nucleic acid synthesis

- ■ Inhibitors of cell wall synthesis

- • Examples
- − Penicillins, cephalosporins, bacitracin, vancomycin, carbapenems, monobactams

- • Mechanisms of action
- − Penicillins and cephalosporins disrupt the cross-linking of peptidoglycan by inhibiting the enzyme transpeptidase; involved in formation of cross-links between the side chains of peptidoglycan
- − Penicillins and cephalosporins also act by binding to penicillin binding proteins to cause activation of autolysis
- − Vancomycin prevent cross-linking of peptidoglycan by binding to D-Ala-D-Ala of cell wall precursor

- • Spectrum of activity
- − Penicillins and cephalosporins are broad spectrum
- − Bacitracin and vancomycin attack gram-positive bacteria
- − The four drugs are bacteriocidal

- Resistance
- Since most of the drugs in this class are β-lactam drugs, bacteria which produce β-lactamase enzyme are able to open their β-lactam ring and abolish their antibacterial effect

- Inhibitors of cell membrane function

- Example: Polymyxin B and colistin

- Mechanism of action
- Polymyxin B and colistin have detergent-like action; they interact with lipopolysaccharide of gram-negative bacteria membrane, to cause increased membrane permeability and decreased osmotic integrity

- Spectrum of activity
- Polymyxin B and colistin attack gram-negative bacteria
- They are bacteriocidal

- Side effect: they are nephrotoxic

- Inhibitors of protein synthesis

- Example
- Aminoglycosides, tetracycline, macrolides, chloramphenicol

- Mechanisms of action
- Aminoglycosides (gentamicin, streptomycin, kanamycin etc.) binds irreversibly with 30S ribosomal subunit, causing misreading of mRNA and in turn decrease protein synthesis
- Tetracycline binds reversibly with 30S ribosomal subunit; inhibiting binding of aminoacyl-tRNA to the ribosome

- Macrolides (erythromycin, clarithromycin, azithromycin etc.) binds reversibly with 50S ribosomal subunit, thus inhibits translocation during protein synthesis
- Chloramphenicol binds to the 23S rRNA of 50S ribosomal subunit, thus inhibits transpeptidation during protein synthesis

- **Spectrum of activity**
- Aminoglycosides, tetracycline, and chloramphenicol are broad spectrum
- Macrolides attack gram-positive bacteria
- Aminoglycosides are bacteriocidal
- Macrolides, tetracycline, and chloramphenicol are bacteriostatic

- **Inhibitors of nucleic acid synthesis**

- **Examples: Quinolones, rifampicin, trimethoprim, pyrimethamine, sulphonamides**

- **Mechanism of actions**
- Quinolones block DNA gyrase (i.e. DNA unwinding) thus inhibits DNA replication
- Rifampicin inhibits RNA polymerase; inhibiting RNA synthesis
- Trimethoprim and pyrimethamine inhibit dihydrofolate reductase; the enzyme that reduces dihydrofolate to folate

- **Spectrum of activity**
- Quinolones and rifampicin are broad spectrum and bacteriocidal
- Other classes of antimicrobial agent shall be discussed at the appropriate section

CHAPTER 7: STAPHYLOCOCCUS

- **Introduction**
- The *Staphylococcus* and the *Streptococcus* are the medically important genera of the gram-positive cocci group; though other genera such as the *Micrococcus, Peptococcus* and *Peptostreptococcus* also exist

-

- **General characteristics**
- They are gram-positive cocci, usually arranged as grape-like irregular clusters
- They are non-motile, non-spore forming facultative anaerobes
- They are catalase-positive and oxidase-negative
- They produce exotoxins and are usually unencapsulated
- They are important inhabitants of the skin and mucous membrane

- **Species**
- Of about 40 species present in the genus, only three are of medical importance:
  - *Staphylococcus aureus*
  - *Staphylococcus epidermidis*
  - *Staphylococcus saprophyticus*

❖ STAPHYLOCOCCUS AUREUS
- **Peculiarities of *S. aureus***
- It is coagulase-positive
- It has microcapsule around its cell envelope
- It is β-hemolytic; with a clear zone of hemolysis surrounding its yellow-gray colonies on blood agar plate

- Virulence factors
- *S. aureus* has a myriad of virulence factors, which may account for the wide range of diseases it causes

Antigenic Structures	Enzymes	Exotoxins
Peptidoglycan	Catalase	Hemolysins ($\alpha,\beta,\gamma,$
Teichoic Acid	Hyaluronidase	and δ) Leukocidin
Protein A	Staphylokinase	Exfoliative Toxin
Coagulase	Proteinases	Enterotoxin
Clumping Factor	β-Lactamase	Toxic Shock Syndrome toxin

- Diseases caused by *S. aureus*
- Based on their pathogenesis, *S. aureus* diseases can be grouped into two (table 7.2):
    - Those due to direct invasion of organs
    - Those due to exotoxins

Due to direct invasion of organs	Due to exotoxins
Folliculitis	Food poisoning
Furuncles	Toxic shock syndrome
Impetigo	Scalded skin syndrome
Wound infections	
Pneumonia	
Bacteremia	
Osteomyelitis	
Endocarditis	
Meningitis	
Urinary tract infection	

- Food poisoning
- This is caused by in vivo enterotoxin release or ingestion of enterotoxin contaminated food

36

- The enterotoxin acts directly on the enteric nervous system to stimulate peristalsis
- After a short incubation period (1-8 hrs) nausea, vomiting, and diarrhoea ensue
- It is usually self-limiting, and recovery is rapid

- Toxic shock syndrome (TST)
- This a fatal multi-systemic disease, that occur within 5days of onset of menses in women who use tampons
- Non-menses related type occurs in children or men with staphylococcal wound infection
- It is related to release of TST toxin by TST-associated *S. aureus*
- Patient presents with high fever, of sudden onset, vomiting, diarrhea, myalgia, scarlatiniform rash, and hypotension; with shock, cardiac and renal failure occurring in severe cases

- Scalded skin syndrome
- This is seen in infants, young children and occasionally older age groups, due to infection by exfoliative toxin-producing *S. aureus*
- It is characterised by the detachment of epidermis from the underlying dermis (exfoliation)
- Patient presents with widespread fluid-filled blisters that ruptures easily

- Laboratory diagnosis

- Specimen: pus, sputum, blood, feces, vomitus, food etc.

- Microscopy: Gram positive cocci are seen

- Culture
- **Non-selective media:** - blood agar, nutrient agar, MacConkey's agar

✓ **Selective media:** mannitol salt agar
- On MacConkey's agar, the colonies appears small and pink
- On blood agar, most strains are β-hemolytic; producing a clear zone of hemolysis around their colonies

• Biochemical reactions
- Catalase test – positive
- Coagulase test – positive
- Urea hydrolysis test - positive
- Reduces nitrate to nitrite
- Ferments mannitol

▪ Treatment
- Benzyl penicillin – if strain is sensitive
- Cloxacillin or methicillin - for β-lactamase producing strains
- Vancomycin – for methicillin resistant staphylococcus aureus (MRSA)

❖ STAPHYLOCOCCUS EPIDERMIDIS
- *S. epidermidis* is a coagulase-negative specie
- It inhabit the skin and mucous membrane and thus, a common cause of stitch abscess
- It has predilection for implanted foreign bodies, such as prosthetic valves, shunts, intravascular catheters etc. This is because of its polysaccharide capsule, which mediates its adherence to these structures
- Thus, *S. epidermidis* is the most frequently isolated organism from infected indwelling prosthetic devices
- It also causes endocarditis in intravenous drug abusers and cystitis in people with structural anomalies of the urinary tract

▪ Treatment
- Vancomycin

❖ STAPHYLOCOCCUS SAPROPHYTIICUS
- *S. saprophyticus* like *S. epidermidis* is coagulase-negative
- It is a leading cause of urinary tract infection in sexually active young women

▪ Treatment
- Penicillin

CHAPTER 8: STREPTOCOCCUS

- The genus Streptococcus is another medically important member of the gram-positive cocci group

- **General characteristics**

- They are gram-positive cocci, usually arranged in pairs or chains
- They are non-motile, non-spore forming facultative anaerobes
- They are both catalase and oxidase-negative
- They are nutritionally fastidious organisms
- They live as either commensals, saprophytes or pathogens
- They are fermentative in metabolism; producing lactic acid as the major product

- **Classification**

- The streptococci are so large and heterogeneous that no single system is sufficient to classify them; thus the following schemes are used:
  - Based on serology (Lancefield classification)
  - Based on hemolysis pattern
  - Based on biochemical reactions

- **Based on serology (Lancefield classification)**

- The cell wall of many Streptococci has a carbohydrate called group specific antigen, and this form the basis for their serologic grouping into Lancefield groups:
  - Group A streptococcus: - *Streptococcus pyogenes*
  - Group B streptococcus: - *Streptococcus agalactiae*
  - Group C streptococcus: - *Streptococcus equisimilis*
  - Group F and G streptococci: - *Streptococcus anginosus*
  - Group D streptococcus: - *Streptococcus bovis, S. durans, S. avium*

- Streptococci lacking group specific antigens: - *Streptococcus pneumonia* and viridans streptococci
- Viridans streptococci comprise the following groups of streptococci:
  - Streptococcus mutans group
  - Streptococcus sanguis group
  - Streptococcus salivarius group
  - Streptococcus militis group
  - Streptococcus anginosus-milleri group

▪ **Based on hemolysis pattern**

— Many streptococci are able to hemolyze red blood cells when cultured on sheep blood agar, however the extent to which they hemolyze varies; thus, three types of hemolysis are seen:

- **α-hemolysis:** - incomplete hemolysis, with reduction of hemoglobin, and formation of green pigment
- **β-hemolysis:** - complete hemolysis, with clearing of the blood around the bacterial growth
- **γ-hemolysis:** - no hemolysis

— Group A (*S. pyogenes*) and Group B (*S. agalactiae*) are β-hemolytic

— Group D (*S. bovis, S. durans, S. avium*) are usually α or γ-hemolytic

— *Streptococcus pneumonia* and viridans streptococci are α-hemolytic

▪ **Based on biochemical reactions**

— This is used for species that cannot be grouped by serology

— The biochemical test used include: sugar fermentation reactions, tests for presence of enzymes, tests for susceptibility or resistance to certain chemical agents etc.

❖ GROUP A β-HEMOLYTIC STREPTOCOCCUS (Streptococcus pyogenes)

− *S. pyogenes* possess Lancefield group A antigens, and gives β-hemolysis on blood agar

− It is the most important human pathogen; it is associated with local and systemic invasion and post-infection immunologic disorders.

▪ Virulence factors

− Like *S. aureus, S. pyogenes* has a myriad of virulence factors, which may account for the wide range of diseases

Antigenic Structures	Enzymes	Exotoxins
M-protein Group A antigen T-substance Lipotechoic acid	Streptolysin O Streptolysin S Streptokinase Hyaluronidase Streptodornase (DNase)	Exotoxin A (a.k.a. erythrogenic toxin A) Exotoxin B Exotoxin C

● M-protein

− This is a major virulent factor of *S. pyogenes*

− When absent the organism is not virulent, but will escape phagocytosis

− The protein is heat-stable and acid-stable, but is trypsin-labile

− Immunity to *S. pyogenes* infection is related to the presence of M-protein

− There are up to 150 types of M-protein, thus an individual can have repeated infections with *S. pyogenes*

- Streptolysin O
- A protein that is hemolytically active in the reduced-state and is rapidly inactivated in the presence of oxygen; hence the "O" stands for oxygen-labile
- It is responsible for the hemolysis associated with *S. pyogenes*
- it is antigenic, thus, development of anti-streptolysin O (ASO) antibodies follows *S. pyogenes* infection
- ASO blocks hemolysis by Streptolysin O and it is detectable in recent infection

- Exotoxin A
- This is seen only in few strains of *S. pyogenes*
- It is associated with scarlet fever and streptococcal toxic shock syndrome

- Diseases caused by *S. pyogenes*
- *S. pyogenes* diseases can be conveniently divided into two (table 8.2):
  - Suppurative diseases
  - Non- suppurative diseases

Suppurative diseases	Non-suppurative diseases
Pharyngitis	Rheumatic fever
Pyoderma (impetigo)	Acute glomerulonephritis
Cellulitis	Scarlet fever
Gingivitis	Invasive bacteremia (streptococcal
Necrotizing fasciitis	toxic shock syndrome)
Lymphagitis	
Dental caries	

- Scarlet fever
- This is characterised by fever, pharyngitis, tonsillitis and a red rash

- The rash, caused by exotoxin A , progresses from the trunk and neck to the limbs and face and sometimes followed by desquamation
- Others symptoms include a red or white strawberry tongue, and lines of hyperpigmentation in body creases called Pastia lines

• Laboratory diagnosis
- **Specimen:** - throat swab, pus, blood, serum etc.

✓ **Microscopy**
- Staining of smear of the pus shows single cocci or pairs, which may appear gram-negative; as the cells are no longer viable

✓ **Culture**
❖ Media: - blood agar
- Blood culture will grow *S. pyogenes* within hours to days
- α-hemolytic streptococci may grow slowly, and may require few days to turn positive

✓ **Serologic tests**
- A rise in antibody titres to *S. pyogenes* antigens can be estimated.
- Examples: antibodies to ASO, in respiratory disease, or antibodies to anti-DNase and anti-hyaluronidase, in skin infection, can be estimated for diagnosis

▪ Diseases caused by other streptococcus group

Group	Disease
Group B (*S. agalactiae*)	Neonatal sepsis, meningitis, pneumonia, UTI etc.
Group C and G	Pharyngitis, sinusitis, impetigo, bacteremia, endocarditis etc.
Group D (*S. bovis, S. durans, S. avium*)	Subacute bacterial endocarditis, dental caries, UTI etc.

Streptococcus pneumoniae	Pneumonia, meningitis, bacteremia etc.

- **Treatment**
- For *S. pyogenes*: -   Penicillin G, erythromycin, clindamycin, cephalexin
- For *S. agalactiae*: - Penicillin G, Vancomycin

CHAPTER 9: *NEISSERIA*

- The *Neisseria* is the most important genus of the gram-negative cocci group; though other genera such as the *Moraxella* and *Veillonella* also exist.

■ General characteristics of *Neisseria*

- Neisseria are gram-negative cocci, usually arranged in pairs; thus, called diplococci
- They are kidney-shaped, having flat or concave adjacent edges
- They are non-motile, piliated bacteria that grow best under aerobic condition
- They are oxidase-positive; as they posses the enzyme cytochrome C
- They are rapidly killed by drying, sunlight and many disinfectants

■ Species

Pathogenic species	Non-pathogenic species
N. meningitidis	N. catarrhalis
N. gonorrhoeae	N. lactamica
	N. subflava
	N. sicca

■ Pathogenic species

- They are pathogenic only to human
- They are characteristically found within polymorphonuclear cells
- They are nutritionally fastidious organisms; requiring enriched media for growth
- Their growth is inhibited by free fatty acid and toxic trace metals
- They ferment sugar to produce acid

❖ NEISSERIA GONORRHOEAE

- *Neisseria gonorrhoea*, often called gonococcus, is the specific etiologic agent of gonorrhea.

▪ Peculiarities of *N. gonorrhoeae*
- It is unencapsulated
- It oxidizes only glucose to produce acid
- It is piliated and forms distinctive colonies
- Its endotoxin is a lipo-oligosaccharide
- It has plasmids

▪ Virulence factors

Virulence factor	Function
Pili (fimbrae)	Enhances its attachment to host cells It is antiphagocytic
Por/protein I	Prevents phagolysosome formation; the reason why they are characteristically found within polymorphonuclear cells
Opa/protein II	Involved in attachment to host cells
Lipo-oligosaccharide (LOS)	Responsible for the endotoxic activities of *N. gonorrhoeae* Helps to escape the host immune system (through antigenic mimicry)

❖ GONORRHEA

- Gonorrhea is an highly infectious sexually transmitted disease of human
- It is caused by *N.* gonorrhoeae, which is abundant in the human genital tract

▪ Mode of transmission
- Through unprotected sexual intercourse with infected persons
- Through an infected birth canal in neonates

- Forms of infection
- Genital infection
- Systemic infection

- Genital infection
- The clinical presentation of genital gonorrhoea differs between male and female.

✓ **In male**
- Urethritis and dysuria are the most common presentation in men
- Within 2-6 days of entry, the organisms penetrate the urethral mucous membrane; causing inflammation (acute urethritis)
- There is associated painful urination (dysuria) and mucopurulent discharge from the anterior urethra
- Infection may spread, causing inflammation of the prostate, seminal vesicles, bladder and epididymis
- Involvement of the periurethral tissue, with rupture of the resulting abscesses may lead to formation of the so called "watering can" perineum
- With poor or no treatment, chronic inflammation and healing by fibrosis ensue, leading to urethral stricture and not uncommonly, infertility

✓ **In female**
- Urethritis and cervicitis are the most common presentation in women
- Vaginitis does not usually occur in adults, due to high vaginal acidity
- Infection may spread, causing inflammation of the endometrium, fallopian tubes and ovaries called pelvic

inflammatory disease (PID), which may lead to sterility and ectopic pregnancy
- Rarely, peritonitis may develop, causing inflammation of the peritoneal capsule of the liver and tissue around the liver; called Fitz-Hugh-Curtis syndrome
- Prepubertal females commonly present with vulvovaginitis

✓ **In both sex**
- Rectal inflammation; proctitis may occur, causing purulent anal discharge and tenesmus
- Pharyngitis may occur in adults; due to oral-anal sex practise
- Conjunctivitis may occur due to autoinfection; itching the eye with an infected hand

✓ **In neonates**
- Acute conjunctivitis may occur in neonates born to mothers with genital gonorrhea infection; this is called ophthalmia neonatorum
- Transmission occurs during passage of the fetus through the infected birth canal
- It is a very serious condition that may result in blindness if neglected

▪ **Systemic infection (Gonococcal bacteremia)**
- This is due systemic dissemination of the gonococcus, via the blood stream; it may present as any of the following:
- Gonococcal arthritis
- Gonococcal endocarditis
- Skin lesions
- Gonococcal meningitis (very rarely)

● **Laboratory diagnosis**
- Specimen: - pus, urethral, cervical and eye swab, synovial fluid, blood etc.

✓ **Microscopy**

– Reveals gram-negative diplococci within polymorphonuclear cells

– It is diagnostic in men but unreliable in women

✓ **Culture**

– As the organisms are nutritionally fastidious, and are rapidly killed by drying, specimen should be inoculated immediately after collection, onto an enriched selective media such as:

• Thayer Martins medium (contains vancomycin, colistin and nystatin)

• Modified Thayer Martins medium (content of TM plus trimethoprim)

• Modified New York City medium

– They grow within 48 hours and are identified by being oxidase-positive and utilization of only glucose

▪ Treatment

– **Previously**, it was **penicillin G** but due to the emergence of penicillase producing *N. gonorrhoeae,* we **now** use **ceftriaxone** (a third generation cephalosporin)

– Azithromycin should be used; to treat a possible concomitant chlamydial infection

❖ NEISSERIA MENINGITIDIS

– *Neisseria meningitidis*, often called meningococcus, does not only cause meningitis but also produces a   life-threatening sepsis called meningococcemia

– It is found in the nasopharynx of 5-10% of healthy individuals

▪ Peculiarities of *N. meningitidis*

– It has polysaccharide capsule

– It oxidizes both glucose and maltose to produce acid

- They are piliated but do not form distinctive colonies
- Its endotoxin is a lipopolysaccharide
- It rarely have plasmids

- Virulence factors

Virulence factor	Function
Capsular polysaccharides	It is antiphagocytic It is immunogenic i.e. induces antibody production It is used in classifying *N. meningitidis* into serogroups
Lipopolysaccharide (LPS)	It is responsible for the endotoxic activities of *N. meningitidis*
IgA protease	It cleaves IgA; allowing oropharynx colonization

- Mode of transmission
- Through droplets from patients or asymptomatic carriers
- Transmission is enhanced by close contact and overcrowding

- Disease and pathogenicity
- Human are the only natural hosts for whom meningococci is pathogenic
- The nasopharynx is the portal of entry; where they attach with the aid of pili
- From the nasopharynx, organisms reach the blood stream, producing meningococcemia
- Depending on the organs to which they spread, patient may present with meningitis and or fulminant meningococcemia

- Meningitis
- This is the most common manifestation of meningococcemia
- Onset is usually sudden and patient present with intense headache, vomiting, stiff neck, with rapid progression to coma

- Note that, spread of *N. meningitidis* directly from the nasopharynx into the subarachnoid space, though uncommon, is a cause of meningitis without meningococcemia

- **Fulminant meningococcemia**
- This is a less common but more severe manifestation of meningococcemia
- Patient present with bilateral adrenal hemorrhages, petechial hemorrhages, and fever; accompanied by disseminated intravascular coagulation, hypotension, shock and coma.
- The above is called Waterhouse-Friderichsen syndrome
- Occasionally, chronic meningococcal arthritis and endocarditis may ensue

- **Laboratory Diagnosis**
- Specimen: - blood, cerebrospinal fluid (CSF), nasopharyngeal swab, skin smear

- **Microscopy**
- Gram-stained smears, of the sediment of centrifuged CSF or of petechial aspirate, show gram-negative diplococci within or outside the polymorphonuclear cells

- **Culture**
- The specimen should be inoculated onto modified Thayer Martins medium, immediately after collection
- They are identified by being oxidase-positive and utilization of both glucose and maltose

- **Treatment**
- Penicillin G is the drug of choice
- Chloramphenicol or a third generation cephalosporin (cefotaxime or ceftriaxone) is used in persons allergic to penicillin

CHAPTER 10: AEROBIC GRAM-POSITIVE BACILLI

- This group of bacteria have the common features of being able to retain the purple color of crystal violet dye during Gram staining, and of requiring molecular oxygen for growth

- **Classification**
- Based on their ability to form spores, this group is divided into two (table 10.1):
  - Spore-forming aerobic gram-positive bacilli
  - Nonspore-forming aerobic gram-positive bacilli

Spore-forming AGPB	Nonspore-forming AGPB
Bacillus spp.	*Corynebacterium spp.*
	Listeria spp.
	Erysipelothrix spp.

- ❖ **BACILLUS**
- **General characteristics of *Bacillus spp.***
- They are large gram-positive bacilli, usually arranged in chains
- They are aerobic spore-forming organisms
- They nutritionally non-fastidious
- They are catalase-positive
- Most members are saprophytes
- Some species are motile while others are not motile

- **Endospore of *Bacillus spp.***
- Bacillus species form endospores as a means of survival in adverse environmental conditions
- The endospores are highly resistant to heating, drying, and disinfection.
- They have a low metabolic activity and thus, are able to withstand long period of starvation

- They readily revert back to the vegetative cell once the environmental condition is favourable e.g. when ingested by a susceptible host

▪ Species

Pathogenic species	Saprophytic species
B. anthracis	B. polymyxa
B. cereus	B. subtilis
	B. stearothermophilus

Table 10.2

- Saprophytic Species
- B. polymyxa produces the antibiotic polymyxin
- B. subtilis produces the antibiotic bacitracin
- B. stearothermophilus produce the most heat-resistant spore
- Though uncommon, they are able produce infections such as bacteremia, meningitis etc.

❖ BACILLUS ANTHRACIS

- B. anthracis was first described as a spore-forming organism and the etiology of anthrax by Robert Koch in the year 1876
- It is not only the first bacterium shown to be the cause of a disease, but also the first bacterium to be used in the preparation of an attenuated vaccine (Louis Pasteur in 1881)

▪ Peculiarities of B. anthracis

- They have a characteristic rectangular shape
- They are non-motile, aerobic organism
- Their endospores are centrally located, oval in shape, and highly refractile to light
- Each spore is encapsulated within a capsule made of poly-D-glutamic acid

- Virulence factors

Virulence factor	Function
Capsular polysaccharide	It is antiphagocytic It is a determinant of virulence
Anthrax toxin	It is a complex of three proteins: **protective antigen, edema factor**, and **lethal factor** The three interact, to produce tissue edema and necrosis; leading to patient's death

❖ **ANTHRAX**
- Anthrax is an infectious disease, caused by *B. anthracis*
- It primarily affects herbivores, with humans as incidental hosts; thus, it is a zoonosis

- **Mode of transmission**
- Through ingestion of spores by animals while grazing
- Through contact with infected animals or their products
- Shepherds, butchers, military recruits and wool sorters are especially at risk

- **Disease and Pathogenicity**
- The ingested spores germinate into vegetative cells within the animal, and are shed in discharges from all orifices (mouth, nose, anus etc.)
- The bacilli then sporulate i.e. form spores, which contaminate the environment
- Depending on the route of spore entry, human disease may present as:

- **Cutaneous anthrax**
- This is the commonest form of anthrax, it is caused by spore contamination of open wound

- A pruritic, non-painful lesion appear, which progresses from papule to blister and pustule; with a black area of skin necrosis called eschar
- The eschar is surrounded by a spreading edema (called malignant edema) and induration
- Though it may heal up or become systemic, mortality is generally low

• Pulmonary anthrax (Wool sorters diseases)
- This is a highly mortal form of anthrax, caused by inhalation of the spores
- The spores are transported to regional lymph nodes where they germinate, multiply and release exotoxins
- It is characterised by hemorrhagic inflammation and edema of the mediastinum; causing dyspnea, septicemia, meningitis and shock
- It is an occupational hazard for wool sorters; thus, it is a.k.a. Wool sorters diseases

• Gastrointestinal anthrax
- This is a very rare mortal form of anthrax, acquired by ingestion of uncooked or poorly cooked spore contaminated meat
- Spores are deposited in the intestinal submucosa, ultimately causing massive edema, that may obstruct the intestinal lumen, with hemorrhage and necrosis

▪ Laboratory diagnosis
- Specimen: - exudates, blood, sputum, aspirates, CSF etc.

• Microscopy
- Chains of large gram-positive rods with centrally placed spores are seen

- Culture
- Non-hemolytic gray to white colonies with rough texture and a ground-glass appearance is seen on blood agar plate
- There colonies shows a medusa head appearance on nutrient agar

- Treatment
- Ciprofloxacin
- Penicillin G, with gentamicin or streptomycin has **previously** been used

- Prevention
- Proper disposal and autoclaving of animal waste products
- Vaccination of animals and people at risk of infection

❖ BACILLUS CEREUS
- *B. cereus* is a soil organism that typically causes food poisoning

- Virulence factors
- Heat-labile toxin
- Heat-stable toxin

- Disease and pathogenicity
- *B. cereus* commonly contaminates rice or meats, with its spores
- The spores are not inactivated by cooking the food to 100^0C
- On cooling, the y germinate into the vegetative cells, which then multiply and elaborate enterotoxins onto the food
- Based on the incubation period, two forms of *B. cereus* food poisoning are known.

Early onset (Emetic type)	Late onset (Diarrheal type)
– Has an incubation period of	– Has an incubation period of

1-5 hours	1-24 hours
– Usually follows rice ingestion	– Usually follows meat ingestion
– Characterised by severe vomiting	– Characterised by profuse diarrhea, abdominal pain and cramp

- Note that, besides food poisoning, *B. cereus* is also an important cause of eye infections, such as severe keratitis, endophthalmitis, and panophthalmitis

- **Diagnosis**
- Bacteria concentration of up to 10^5 or more per gram of food is considered diagnostic

- **Treatment**
- Food-borne infections are treated symptomatically e.g. rehydration.
- Serious non-food borne infection should be treated with **vancomycin** or **clindamycin** with or without **aminoglycoside**
- *B. cereus* is resistant to penicillins and cephalosporins

- ❖ CORYNEBACTERIUM
- Various pathogenic and saprophytic species occur within this genus; however, focus will be on the main pathogenic specie, which is *Corynebacterium diphtheria*
- *C. diphtheria*, a.k.a. klebs-loeffler bacillus, is the causative agent of diphtheria

- **Characteristics of *C. diphtheria***
- It is a non-motile nonspore-forming gram-positive bacilli
- It is non-capsulated, having club-shaped ends

- it gives the characteristic Chinese letter appearance during binary fission
- Its metachromatic (Volutin) granules stain deeply using Albert's staining technique
- They grow aerobically on most ordinary media

- Virulence
- The virulence of *C. diphtheria* is due to three factors:
  - Their ability to establish infection
  - Their ability to grow rapidly
  - Their ability to quickly elaborate the diphtheria toxin

- Diphtheria toxin
- This is an exotoxin produced by virulent (lysogenic) strains of *C. diphtheria*
- it inhibits protein synthesis by inactivating a factor (EF-2) required for transfer of polypeptidyl-tRNA to ribosomes
- The abrupt cessation of protein synthesis result in necrosis of the affected cells
- Note that, low iron concentration in the organism increases toxin production

- Classification
- Based on their ability to elaborate the diphtheria toxin, strains of *C. diphtheria* are sub-divided into two:
  - Toxigenic strains
  - Non-toxigenic strains

- Mode of transmission
- Through direct contact with secretions of infected persons or carriers, and through droplets

- Pathogenesis
- Following entry, the bacilli grow and multiply on the mucosa of nasopharynx, but they do not penetrate deeply into the underlying tissue or blood
- They in turn elaborate the powerful diphtheria toxin, which is absorbed into the mucosa; causing inflammation and destruction of the mucosa
- In turn, a grayish pseudomembrane, composed of fibrin, *C. diphtheria,* erythrocytes and leukocytes is formed over the tonsils, pharynx, and larynx
- The exotoxin diffuses throughout the body with predilection for the heart, nerves, liver, kidney and adrenals.

- Clinical features
- Sore throat
- Fever
- Prostration
- Dyspnea
- Neuropathy
- Myocarditis and cardiac arrhythmias

- Laboratory diagnosis
- Specimen: - swabs of throat, nasal cavity or other lesions

- Microscopy
- Gram-positive, nonspore-forming colonies are seen

- Culture
- ❖ Media: - blood agar, Loeffler's serum slope, serum tellurite medium etc.
- Growth on the above media is rapid; within 12-18 hours
- Demonstrate for Volutin granule using Albert's staining technique

- Note that, specific treatment should never be delayed for laboratory report if clinical picture is strongly suggestive of diphtheria

- Treatment
- **Penicillin, erythromycin**; to arrest toxin production by the remaining bacteria
- **Diphtheria antitoxin**; to neutralize the remaining toxins

- ❖ LISTERIA
- This genus is named after Joseph Lister, the English pioneer of sterile surgery, in 1940
- The main human pathogen in the genus is *L. monocytogenes;* the causative agent of listerosis

- Characteristics of *L. monocytogenes*
- It is a short, gram-positive, nonspore-forming bacilli
- It has 4 flagella and thus actively motile; at 25^0C but not at 37^0C
- It is catalase-positive and β-hemolytic on blood agar
- It produces acid without gas from utilization of carbohydrate

- Pathogenesis
- *L. monocytogenes* enters the body through the gastrointestinal tract
- It adhere to the host's intestinal cells via it adhesion proteins
- Though they are phagocytised, they have mechanisms of escaping out of the phagocytes
- They produce disease by release of exotoxins in form of hemolysins

- Clinical presentation

• Meningo-encephalitis
  - This most commonly occur in immunosuppressed patients
  - It produces suppurative meningitis with mostly mononuclear cells in the CSF; causing a monocytosis in the blood, hence the name "monocytogenes"

• Granulomatosis infantiseptica
  - This is a generalised listeriosis that occurs in newborn, due to an inutero transmission of the organisms from an asymptomatic mother
  - Neonatal sepsis ensue, causing extensive focal necrosis especially in the liver and spleen
  - Death occur before or shortly after delivery, in early-onset type, and around third week of life, in late-onset type

- Laboratory diagnosis
  - Isolation of the organism in cultures of blood and cerebrospinal fluid (CSF)

- Treatment
  - **Ampicillin** with **erythromycin** or intravenous **co-trimoxazole**

❖ ERYSIPELOTHRIX
  - The most important specie is *E. rhusiopathiae*, which causes erysipeloid in humans

- Characteristics of *E. rhusiopathiae*
  - It is a slender non-motile nonspore-forming gram-positive bacilli
  - It produces acid without gas from utilization of carbohydrate
  - They catalase- and oxidase-negative

- ▪ Disease and Pathogenesis
- − People obtain *E. rhusiopathiae* through direct inoculation from animals or their products
- − Fishermen, fish handlers, butchers etc. are especially at risk of infection

- • Erysipeloid
- − After an incubation period of 2-7 days, pain and swelling occurs at the site, usually the finger
- − The lesion is raised and violaceous in color, without pus formation
- − It may be accompanied by fever and arthritis symptoms
- − Rarely, extension of the lesion with bacteremia and endocarditis may occur

- ▪ Treatment
- − Penicillin G

CHAPTER 11: ANAEROBIC GRAM-POSITIVE BACILLI

- This group of bacteria have the common features of being able to retain the purple color of crystal violet dye, and of being able to grow only in the absence of molecular oxygen

▪ Classification
- Based on their ability to form spores, this group is divided into two
  • Spore-forming anaerobic gram-positive bacilli
  • Nonspore-forming anaerobic gram-positive bacilli

Spore-forming AnGPB	Nonspore-forming AnGPB
Clostridium spp.	Propionibacterium spp. Bifidobacterium spp. Lactobacillus spp.

❖ CLOSTRIDIUM
▪ General characteristics of Clostridium spp.
- They are spore-forming anaerobic gram-positive bacilli
- Most species are motile (C. perfringens is not motile)
- Pathogenic species produce highly potent exotoxins or enzymes
- They possess peritrichous flagellation but generally lacks tissue invasion
- They may produce saccharolytic and or proteolytic effect

• Endospore of Clostridium spp.
- Clostridium spp. form endospores as a means of survival in adverse conditions
- The spores are usually wider than the diameter of the rods in which they are formed

- They may be centrally, subterminally, or terminally placed, depending on the specie
- They are resistant to physical and chemical agents, but are destroyed by autoclaving
- They revert to the vegetative cell once the condition is favourable e.g. anaerobic condition

■ Pathogenic species and their associated disease

Specie	Disease
C. tetani	Tetanus
C. perfringens	Gas gangrene
C. botulinum	Botulism
C. difficile	Pseudomembranous colitis

❖ CLOSTRIDIUM TETANI (Tetanus)

- C. tetani is the causative agent of tetanus; an acute paralytic illness characterized by repeated painful muscle spasms, hypertonia and dysautonomia

■ Peculiarities of C. tetani
- It is a motile, obligate-anaerobic gram-positive bacilli
- Its endospores are located terminally, giving it a drum-stick appearance
- Its endospores are widely distributed; in soil, dust, rusted metals, animal feces etc.

■ Toxins of C. tetani
- Two exotoxins are produced by C. tetani: tetanospasmin and tetanolysin

Tetanospasmin	Tetanolysin
A potent neurotoxin, which is primarily responsible for	It produces red cell lysis Its role in the

the features of tetanus. It is a plasmid encoded 150 kDa protein It acts by inhibiting the inhibitory interneurons of skeletal muscles in the spinal cord It is lethal in extremely small amounts	pathogenesis of tetanus is not completely understood

- **Mode of infection**
- Through contamination of open wounds with spores of *C. tetani*
- Wounds on the sole, umbilicus, ear, and the female genitals are common routes of entry
- Note that, the portal of entry is not identifiable in about 30% of patients

- **Pathogenesis**
- Under anaerobic condition, the spores germinate into vegetative cells, which release exotoxins (tetanospasmin and tetanolysin) into the necrotic tissue
- Tetanospasmin enters the motor neurons, within the wound, and travels retrogadely within the axons of the nerves, to reach the anterior horn cells of the spinal cord and brainstem
- Within the spinal cord and brain stem, tetanospasmin cleaves the protein synaptobrevin, which is involved in binding of vesicles containing inhibitory neurotransmitters, glycine and γ-amino butyric acid(GABA), to the cell membrane for release
- As a result, Glycine and GABA are not released; leading to the loss of inhibitory actions of the higher centers on motor and autonomic neurons of the spinal cord and brainstem

- Thus, this disinhibited neuron continuously discharge impulses to the muscles, causing hyperexcitability, spasms and hypertonia

- Clinical features

Clinical feature	Explanation
Trismus (first symptom)	Patient is unable to open the mouth, due to spasm of the masseter muscle. It is a.k.a. lock jaw
Risus sardonicus	Grinning expression due to spasm of muscles of facial expression. It is a.k.a. devil's smile
Opisthotonos	Extreme hyperextension of the body; with head and heels bent backward and the trunk bowed forward, due to generalised muscle spasm
Laryngospasm	Spasm of laryngeal muscles, causing aspiration, asphyxia, and death
Dysphagia Hydrophobia Drooling of saliva	All result from spasm of esophageal muscle
Fever Tachycardia Fluctuations in blood pressure Excessive sweating Cardiac arrhythmias	These are features of dysautonomia, and they are poor prognostic factors

- Note that while the patient experiences the above, consciousness is usually preserved
- The usual causes of death in tetanus include exhaustion, laryngospasm, pulmonary thromboembolism or cardiac arrhythmia

- Diagnosis
- Diagnosis is based on clinical picture and history of wound (if available) supported by laboratory findings:
- ❖ Specimen: - wound exudates, ear and umbilical wound swab, high vaginal swab etc.

- Microscopy
- Shows gram-positive bacilli with terminal spores

- Culture
- ❖ Media: - blood agar, Robertson cooked meat medium
- It gives greyish semi-transparent swarming colonies on blood agar
- It produces only proteolytic effect on Robertson cooked meat medium

- Treatment
- Intramuscular administration of 10,000 units of anti-tetanus serum to neutralize toxins that as not fix to nerve tissue
- Control of spasms and continuous sedation with phenobarbitone, chlorpromazine, and diazepam
- Elimination of residual clostridial infection through wound debridement
- Administer **metronidazole** to inhibit growth of *C. tetani,* and prevent further toxin release
- Adequate food and calorie intake through a nasogastric tube
- Optimal nursing and general supportive care e.g. intravenous fluids, intranasal oxygen etc.
- Immunization of survivors prior to discharge
- ❖ Penicillin should be avoided because it acts like competitive GABA antagonist; thus, potentiate the disinhibition

❖ **CLOSTRIDIUM PERFRINGENS (Gas gangrene)**
- By definition, gas gangrene is a rapidly spreading necrosis accompanied by gas bubble formation in an injured soft tissue
- *C. perfringens* account for about 90% of severe cases of gas gangrene
- Other causative species are: *C. novyi, C. septicum, C. histolyticum, C. bifermentans* etc.

▪ Peculiarities of *C. perfringens*
- It is a non-motile gram-positive bacilli
- Its endospores are subterminally placed
- It does not form spores when grown on laboratory media
- It is subdivided into five strains (A-E)

▪ Toxins and enzymes of *C. perfringens*

Toxins and enzymes	Characteristics
α-toxin	The most important of all toxins Produced by all strains (A-E) It is a lecithinase; which breaks down lecithin of the cell membrane
Enterotoxin	Causes food poisoning; especially meat dishes
β-toxin	Produced by *C. perfringens* type C Causes enteritis necroticans
Hyaluronidase	A collagenase that digests collagen of subcutaneous tissue and muscle

▪

▪ Pathogenesis
- Spores gain entry into dirty wounds from soil, or into surgical wounds from patients flora
- Under anaerobic condition, the spores germinate into vegetative cells
- The cells multiply and ferment tissue carbohydrates to produce gases (H_2 and CO_2)

- The distension of tissue with gas, which interfere with blood supply and the secretion of α-toxins and hyaluronidase, favour rapid spread of infection
- Ultimately, tissue necrosis extends rapidly, leading to severe toxaemia and death

- Clinical features
- This is conveniently divided into two: local signs of gas gangrene and features of toxemia

Local signs of gas gangrene	Features of toxemia
Myositis	Severe hemolysis
Myonecrosis	Jaundice
Edema	Acute renal failure
Crepitations; due to gas accumulation	Shock
Discoloration of overlying skin	Death

- Laboratory diagnosis
- ❖ Specimen: - pus, wound swab, blood etc.

- Microscopy
- Shows gram-positive bacilli with subterminal spores

- Culture
- ❖ Media: - blood agar, Robertson cooked meat (RCM) medium
- It produces hemolytic non-swarming colonies on blood agar
- It produces both proteolytic and saccharolytic effects on RCM medium

- Treatment
- Wound debridement (to remove necrotized tissue)
- Polyvalent antiserum (against exotoxins)

- Hyperbaric O (since the organisms are obligate anaerobes)
- Antibiotics (penicillin, metronidazole, gentamicin)
- Treat features of toxaemia

❖ **CLOSTRIDIUM BOTULINUM (Botulism)**
- *C. botulinum* is the causative agent of botulism
- Botulism is an acute potentially lethal neurologic disorder caused by ingestion of food contaminated with botulinum toxin

▪ **Peculiarities of *C. botulinum***
- It is an obligate anaerobic gram-positive bacilli
- Its endospores are subterminally placed
- The spores are extremely resistant to destruction, and can survive for 30 yrs or more!

● **Botulinum toxin**
- Botulinum toxin is the most poisonous substance known to man
- Seven antigenic varieties of the toxin are known (A-G)

▪ **Clinical forms of botulism**
- **Infant botulism**: caused by ingestion of spore contaminated food
- **Food borne botulism**: caused by ingestion of toxin contaminated food
- **Wound botulism:** caused by spore contamination of wound

▪ **Pathogenesis**
- The toxin is absorbed from the gut mucosa or wound into the blood stream

- It then binds irreversibly to receptors on the presynaptic membranes of peripheral motor neurons and cranial nerves
- The light chain of the toxin then cleaves the SNARE proteins, which are responsible for binding of acetylcholine containing vesicles to the presynaptic membrane for release
- As a result, acetylcholine is not released into the synaptic cleft, neurotransmission does not occur, and flaccid paralysis ensue

- **Clinical features**
- Double or blurred vision
- Drooping eyelids
- Dysphagia
- Dry mouth
- Speech difficulty
- Muscle weakness
- Respiratory failure (common cause of death)

- **Diagnosis**
- ❖ Specimen: - ingested food, stool, blood

- **Microscopy**
- Shows gram-positive bacilli with subterminal spores

- **Culture**
- ❖ Media: - blood agar, Robertson cooked meat (RCM)medium
- It produces transparent swarming hemolytic colonies on blood agar
- It produces both proteolytic and saccharolytic effects on RCM medium

- **Treatment**
- Fluid and electrolyte support
- Respiratory support

- Polyvalent antitoxin
- Antibiotic therapy is indicated in infantile botulism, as live organisms were ingested

❖ *CLOSTRIDIUM DIFFICILE* (Pseudomembranous colitis)
- *C. difficile* is a strict anaerobic gram-positive spore-forming bacilli that exist as normal flora in the colon of infants and some adults

• Virulence factors
- Toxin A – an enterotoxins
- Toxin B – a cytotoxin

▪ Pathogenesis
- Pseudomembranous colitis usually follows a long course of broad spectrum antibiotic therapy especially ampicillin, clindamycin and fluoroquinolones
- The antibiotics destroy the normal gut commensals and preserve *C. difficile*
- *C. difficile* in turn overgrow and elaborates their toxins; causing inflammatory response and formation of pseudomembranes over the necrotic intestinal wall

▪ Clinical features
- Diarrhea or dysentery
- Hemorrhage; which may be severe enough to cause death
- Abdominal cramps
- Fever

▪ Laboratory diagnosis
- Detection of one or both *C. difficile* toxins in stool is diagnostic

- Also by endoscopic observation of pseudomembranes or microabscesses

- Treatment
- Discontinue the offending antibiotic, and orally give either **metronidazole** or **vancomycin**

CHAPTER 12: ENTEROBACTERIACEAE

- Enterobacteriaceae is a large family of gram-negative, facultatively anaerobic rods
- They exist naturally in the intestines of man and animal; thus, are otherwise called coliforms
- They, along with staphylococci and streptococci, are among the commonest cause of bacteria diseases

- **General characteristics of Enterobacteriaceae**
- They are gram-negative facultative anaerobes
- They grow readily and rapidly on simple media
- They are either motile with peritrichous flagella or non-motile
- They are catalase-positive and oxidase-negative
- They ferment glucose to form acid, often with gas production
- They reduces nitrate to nitrite

- **Classification**
- The genera under the family enterobacteriaceae have been classified base on several criteria, but only three shall be discussed:
- Based on ability to ferment lactose
- Based on biochemical reactions
- Based on motility

- **Base on ability to ferment lactose**

Rapid lactose fermenters	Slow lactose fermenters	Non-lactose fermenters
Escherichia	Citrobacter	Salmonella
Enterobacter	Serratia	Proteus
Klebsiella	Providencia	Shigella
	Edwardsiella	
	Arizona	
	Erwinia	

- Base on biochemical reactions

Biochemical Test	Escher ichia	Kleb siella	Entero bacter	Citrob acter	Prot eus	Salmo nella	Shig ella
Indole test	+	-	-	-	-	-	-
Methyl red	+	-	-	+	+	+	+
Citrate test	-	+	+	+	v	+	-
Voges-Proskauer test	-	+	+	-	-	-	-

+ (positive for the test) - (negative for the test) v (variable)

- Based on motility
- All genera under the family enterobacteriaceae are motile except *Shigella* and *Klebsiella* which are non-motile

- Antigenic structure
- Enterobacteriaceae generally have three main antigens: O-, K-, and H-antigens
- O-antigens are part of lipopolysaccharide (LPS) and are resistant to both heat and alcohol
- K-antigens are mostly polysaccharides; *E. coli* uses it in attachment to cells, prior to invasion
- H-antigens are located on flagella, and are denatured by both heat and alcohol; Since *Shigella* and *Klebsiella* lack flagella, they also lack this antigens

❖ ESCHERICHIA COLI
- *E. coli* is the principal specie of the genus *Escherichia*, and a common facultative organism of human and animal intestines
- Although only few pathogenic strains exist, they are part of the most frequent cause of urinary tract infection (UTI), diarrhea, neonatal meningitis and pneumonia

- Peculiarities of *E. coli*
- It is positive for indole and methyl red test
- It is negative for citrate and Voges-Proskauer test
- It produces hemolysis on blood agar
- It is motile with peritrichous flagella

❖ **DISEASES CAUSED BY *E. COLI***

▪ Diarrhea

- As a pathogen, *E. coli* is best known for its ability to cause diarrhea
- Based on the characteristic virulence property with which it causes the diarrhea, five classes (virotypes) of *E. coli* are known:

- Enterotoxigenic *E. coli* (ETEC)
- ETEC causes traveller's diarrhea and infantile diarrhea
- It produces heat-labile toxin (LT) that stimulates Cl^- secretion and inhibits Na^+ reabsorption
- It produces heat-stable toxin (ST) which increases fluid secretion
- The gut lumen becomes distended with fluid, causing hypermotility and in turn diarrhea

- Enteropathogenic *E. coli* (EPEC)
- EPEC is a leading cause of infantile diarrhea in developing countries
- They adhere to intestinal cells and destroy the microvilli; a mechanism called "attachment and effacing of cells"
- Diarrhea is believed to be due to moderate invasion of intestinal cells and interference with normal signal transduction; rather than being toxin-mediated

- **Enteroinvasive *E. coli* (EIEC)**
  - It is a common cause of diarrhea among children in and travellers to developing countries
  - The disease is very similar to shigellosis, i.e. involve invasion and destruction of intestinal epithelial cells; no toxin is produced

- **Enteroaggregative *E. coli* (EAEC)**
  - They cause chronic diarrhea in children of developing countries
  - They do not invade or cause inflammation in the intestinal mucosa
  - Diarrhea is due to release of heat-stable-like toxin (ST-like) and hemolysin

- **Enterohemorrhagic *E. coli* (EHEC)**
  - This is the commonest strain producing disease in developed countries
  - They primarily cause hemorrhagic colitis (bloody diarrhea) which may progress to fatal hemolytic-uremic syndrome
  - They are characterised by production of Shiga toxins a.k.a. verotoxin
  - Serotype 0157:H7 is the prototypic EHEC and is the serotype most often implicated in illness world wide

- **Urinary tract infection (UTI)**
  - *E. coli* is the commonest cause of UTI, with most infections originating from the colon
  - Uropathogenic *E. coli* are characterised by possession of pili, with which they migrate up into the urethra to infect the bladder (cystitis) and at times the kidney (pyelonephritis)
  - Patient present with increased urinary frequency, dysuria, hematuria, pyuria, and possibly bacteremia and sepsis

- Meningitis
- Next to group β-hemolytic *streptococci*, *E. coli* is commonest cause of meningitis in infants
- About 75% of *E. coli* causing meningitis bears the K1 antigen

- Sepsis
- *E. coli* is commonest cause of gram-negative sepsis
- Newborn are especially predisposed as they lack IgM antibodies

❖ **KLEBSIELLA PNEUMONIAE**
- *K. pneumoniae* is among the top ten pathogens responsible for hospital-acquired infections

- Peculiarities of *K. pneumoniae*
- It is encapsulated; thus, has K-antigens and O-antigens
- It lacks flagella; thus, lacks H-antigens

- Diseases Caused By *K. Pneumoniae*
- Pneumonia
- Urinary tract infection (in hospitalized patients on catheter)
- Sepsis (next to *E. coli*)

- K. pneumoniae Pneumonia
- Hospitalized patients and alcoholics are especially prone to *K. pneumoniae* pneumonia
- It is characterised by thick bloody sputum (in about 50% of patients)
- The sputum gives a red currant jelly appearance (the color of O-antigen)
- Mortality rate is high despite antibiotic therapy

❖ **PROTEUS MIRABILIS**

- *P. mirabilis* move very actively by means of peritrichous flagella; thus, its colonies coalesce and cover the growth plate (swarming) rather than as distinct round colonies.
- It characteristically breaks down urea into ammonia and CO_2
- It is not pathogenic until it exit the gastrointestinal tract
- It causes UTI, and the urine sample reveals alkaline pH, due to its high ammonia component
- Besides UTI, it also causes pneumonia in debilitated or immunocompromised patients

▪ **Diagnosis of E. coli, K. pneumoniae and P. mirabilis**

❖ Specimen: - urine, blood, pus, cerebrospinal fluid, sputum etc.

● **Microscopy**

- Members of these genera are morphologically similar, so microscopy may not be too helpful
- Presence of large capsule is suggestive of Klebsiella

● **Culture**

- Specimens are plated on both blood agar and differential media
- On differential medial, various biochemical tests is performed for identification

▪ **Treatment**

- The sulphonamides, ampicillin, cephalosporins, fluoroquinolones, and aminoglycosides have marked antibacterial effect against the coliforms, however, laboratory test for antibiotic susceptibility is essential

❖ **SHIGELLA**

- The genus *Shigella* consists of four pathogenic species:
- *S. dysenteriae* (produces the most severe disease)

- *S. flexneri*
- *S. boydii*
- *S. sonnei* (produces the most mild disease)

- ▪ **Peculiarities of *Shigella***
- They are facultative anaerobes but grow best aerobically
- They lack flagella; thus, lack H-antigens
- They are non-lactose fermenters except *S. sonnei*
- They ferment glucose to form acid, but rarely produce gas
- They usually produce hydrogen sulphide (H_2S)
- Their infection are almost always confined to the gastrointestinal tract

- ● Shiga toxin
- This is an heat-labile exotoxin formed by *S. dysenteriae* type 1 (Shiga bacillus) and EHEC
- The toxin is both enterotoxic and neurotoxic
- It has two subunits: A and B; the **B** subunit **b**inds to the host cell membrane glycolipids, while the **A** subunit is internalised for **a**ction.
- The A subunit act by binding to 28S ribosomal RNA (of the 60S ribosomal subunit) to disrupt protein synthesis, leading eventually to death of intestinal cell

- ▪ **Pathogenesis of *Shigella* dysentery**
- *Shigella spp.* enter the host via the mouth, and because they are genetically configured to survive low pH, they make it through the gastric acid barrier
- They invade the microfold (M) cells of the intestines, especially of the sigmoid colon and rectum, penetrating the lamina propria
- Within the lamina propria, they encounter and are ingested by resident macrophages

- They multiply within the macrophages and release daughter cells by triggering apoptosis
- Viable shigellae released from the dead macrophages invade the basolateral surface of the colonic epithelium, spread from cell-to-cell and provoke the synthesis of IL-8
- IL-8 induces neutrophil migration into the intestinal lumen through the wall
- Neutrophil migration destroys the intestinal wall tight-junctions, allowing for further *Shigella* invasion and exacerbates inflammation
- Consequently, mucosal ulcerations and characteristic dysenteric small-volume stools (consisting of mucus, cellular debris, neutrophil exudates, and blood) are produced
- In addition, *S. dysenteriae* type 1 has the ability to elaborate the Shiga toxin, which inhibit protein synthesis in the cells and may lead to extraintestinal complications, including hemolytic-uremic syndrome and death
✓ Note that, invasion of the colonic mucosa, and cell-to-cell spread of infection are essential steps the pathogenesis

- **Clinical features**
- Sudden onset of **abdominal pain**, **fever**, and **watery diarrhea**
- About a day later, feces becomes less watery but contains **mucous** and **blood**
- Defecation is accompanied by **straining** and **tenesmus**; causing **lower abdominal pain**
- In 50% of cases fever and diarrhea subside in 2-5 days; however, the fluid loss and electrolyte derangement may lead to **dehydration**, **acidosis** and even **death**

- **Laboratory diagnosis**
❖ Specimen: - fresh stool, mucus flecks, rectal swabs

- Culture
- Colorless (lactose-negative) colonies that do not produce hydrogen sulphide, that produce acid but not gas and are non-motile should be subjected to agglutination by *Shigella* antisera.

- Treatment
- Ciprofloxacin, ampicillin, doxycycline, co-trimoxazole are all effective

❖ SALMONELLA
- The genus *Salmonella*, like the *Shigella* is not considered as part of the normal intestinal flora as it is primarily pathogenic.
- They account for foodborne illnesses such as typhoid fever and gastroenteritis

- Peculiarities of *Salmonella*
- They are usually motile with peritrichous flagella
- They are non-lactose fermenters
- They ferment glucose to form acid, and sometimes gas
- They usually produce hydrogen sulphide (H_2S)
- They are resistant to bile salt

- Antigenic structure
- Members of the genus *Salmonella* have three antigenic structures:
  - O- antigen – somatic antigen
  - H- antigen – flagellar antigen
  - Vi- antigen – capsular antigen

- Species
- The genus *Salmonella* comprises two species: *S. bongori* and *S. enterica*

- *S. enterica* consists of six subspecies, which are separable into about 2400 serotypes on the basis of their antigenic structures
- However, only four serotypes can cause enteric fever; they include:
  - *Salmonella* Paratyphi A (serogroup A)
  - *Salmonella* Paratyphi B (serogroup B)
  - *Salmonella* Choleraesuis (serogroup C1)
  - *Salmonella* Typhi (serogroup D) – commonest cause

❖ **TYPHOID FEVER**

- Typhoid fever, also known as enteric fever, is an acute potentially fatal multisystemic illness, primarily caused by *Salmonella* Typhi (serogroup D), characterized by fever, malaise, diffuse abdominal pain, and constipation

- **Mode of transmission**
- Through ingestion of food contaminated with feces of patient or chronic carrier
- Direct anal-oral inoculation of organisms (rare)
- The mean infective dose is 10^5-10^8 salmonellae
- Incubation period is 10-14 days

- **Pathogenesis of typhoid fever**
- Following ingestion of the organisms with food or water, they pass down into the intestines
- Within the intestine, they enter into the microfold (M) cells, macrophages and lymphocytes within the Peyer's patches of the ileum; sensitizing this lymphoid tissues in the process.
- Via the macrophages, the organisms are transported to the mesenteric lymph nodes; where they multiply, and enter the blood stream, via the cisterna chyli and the thoracic duct **(primary bacteremia)**

- The organisms are rapidly cleared from the blood by the reticulo-endothelial (RE) cells especially the Kupffer cells of the liver
- Within the RE cells, the organisms multiply rapidly, causing rupture of the RE cells and massive release of the organisms into the blood stream again **(secondary bacteremia)**
- Via the gallbladder, the organisms re-enter the intestine (with bile) and reach the previously sensitized Peyer's patches
- Hypersensitivity reaction results, causing extensive necrosis of the Peyer's patches and formation of oval longitudinal ulcers on the anti-mesenteric border of the intestine
- Separation of the sloughs may cause severe hemorrhage, or perforation of the intestinal wall

- Clinical features

First week	Second week	Third week	Fourth week
Fever (step-ladder)	Fever (plateaus) Features of first week progress Splenomegaly	Typhoid state (apathy, confusion, psychosis)	Fever subsides Mental state and abdominal distension
Abdominal pain Constipation (commoner)		Typhoid facie Myocarditis	improve
Diarrhea Dry cough Headache		Unarousable coma	Improvement in clinical status
Rose spots (on the chest)		Green pea-soup diarrhea Death	

- Laboratory diagnosis
- ❖ Specimen: - blood, stool, urine, bone marrow, rose spot etc.

- Culture
- ❖ Media: - MacConkey's agar, salmonella-shigella (SS) agar, Hektoen enteric agar etc.
- − *Salmonella* Typhi appear as non-lactose fermenting, discrete raised colonies
- − They are motile and oxidase-negative
- − Bone marrow culture is the most sensitive (about 90%) and is not affected by previous antibiotic therapy

- Serology
- − Detects the antibody produced against the *Salmonella* Typhi antigens in patient's serum
- − Examples are: Widal's test, enzyme-linked immunosorbent assay (ELISA)

- Polymerase chain reaction
- − Done using *Salmonella* Typhi as primers
- − It is very sensitive and highly specific, but expensive and not readily available

- Full blood count
- − Anemia
- − Neutropenia
- − Lymphocytosis
- − Thrombocytopenia

- Treatment
- − 1948-1970s – chloramphenicol
- − 1970s-1989 – ampicillin and co-trimoxazole
- − Currently – **Ciprofloxacin, Ofloxacin**, or **Ceftriaxone**

CHAPTER 13: GRAM-NEGATIVE COCCOBACILLI (HAEMOPHILUS, BORDETELLA AND BRUCELLA)

- This is a group of very short gram-negative rod-shaped bacteria
- The three genera, which make up this group are:
  - *Haemophilus*
  - *Bordetella*
  - *Brucella*

❖ HAEMOPHILUS

- General characteristics of *Haemophilus spp*
- They are small, rod-shaped gram-ve bacteria
- They are normal inhabitants of the upper respiratory tract but few are pathogenic
- They require enriched media, containing blood or its derivatives, for growth; this because blood is rich in X factor (hemin) and V factor (nicotinamide adenine dinucleotide)

- Pathogenic species and their associated disease

Specie	Disease
H. influenzae	Meningitis, epiglottitis etc.
H. ducreyi	Chancroid
H. influenzae biogroup aegypticus	Purulent conjunctivitis and purpuric fever
H. parainfluenzae	Infective endocarditis and urethritis

❖ HAEMOPHILUS INFLUENZAE
- Peculiarities of *H. influenza*
- It is a non-motile, gram-ve bacilli, occurring in pairs or short chains
- It is an aerobe, but can grow as a facultative anaerobe

- It does not grow on sheep blood agar except in the vicinity of staphylococci, which release V-factor; this is called "satellite phenomenon"
- Most strains are unencapsulated

- **Antigenic structures**

- **Polysaccharide capsule**
- This is the major determinant of virulence in *H. influenzae*
- It is anti-phagocytic in a non-immune host, and is protective against complement-mediated lysis
- Based on the type of antigens on the capsule, *H. influenza* can be divided into six types (a-f)
- *H. influenza* type b, is the most virulent, and its capsular antigens is polyribose-ribitol phosphate (PRP)
- Unencapsulated strains, like those found in the upper respiratory tract, are less virulent

- **IgA Protease**
- *H. influenzae* produces IgA Protease which degrades secretory IgA of the respiratory mucosa; thus, enhancing its attachment

- **Others**
- Lipopolysaccharides (Endotoxins) and somatic antigens (present on its outer membrane)

- **Diseases and pathogenicity**
- Naturally acquired diseases, caused by *H. influenzae*, occur only in humans
- Children between 5 months-5 years, the aged, and debilitated people are especially susceptible to *H. influenzae* infection, due to reduced level of immunity

- Non-capsulated strains generally cause non-invasive infections, while the capsulated strains cause invasive infections (table 13.2)

H. influenza type b	Nontypeable H. influenza
Meningitis	Chronic bronchitis
Epiglottitis	Otitis media
Pneumonia	Sinusitis
Cellulitis	Conjunctivitis
Septic arthritis	
All diseases caused by nontypeable H. influenzae (to a lesser extent)	

- Laboratory diagnosis
- ❖ Specimen: - nasopharyngeal swabs, pus, blood, sputum, CSF etc.

- Microscopy
- They are seen as very small gram-negative coccobacilli, with no specific arrangement.

- Culture
- ❖ Media: - Chocolate agar or blood agar; in a CO_2-enriched incubator
- Flat, grayish brown colonies are seen on chocolate agar after 24 hours
- It is positive for both catalase and oxidase tests
- It grows on blood agar only when the colonies of staphylococci are present to supply the V-factor (satellite phenomenon)
- It is differentiated from the related gram-negative bacilli by its requirements for X and V factors and by its lack of hemolysis on blood agar

- Note that, diagnosis is considered confirmed when the organism is isolated from sterile body sites such as blood and CSF

- **Latex Agglutination Test (LAT)**
- This is a more sensitive method for diagnosis of *H. influenzae* infection, as it relies on antigen detection rather than viable bacteria.
- It is quicker than culture, and the results are not affected by prior antibiotic therapy

- **Polymerase Chain Reaction**
- PCR has been proven to be more sensitivity and highly specific than LAT and culture

- **Treatment**
- **Cefotaxime**, **ceftriaxone**, **ampicillin** and **ciprofloxacin** are all effective
- Note that some strains of *H. influenzae* (about 20%) produce β-lactamase and are thus, resistant to ampicillin (a penicillin derivative)

- **Prevention**
- *H. influenza* type b disease can be prevented by administration of **Haemophilus b conjugate vaccine** to children

❖ **HAEMOPHILUS DUCREYI**
- *H. ducreyi* is the causative agent of chancroid a.k.a. soft chancre
- Chancroid is a sexually transmitted disease characterized by painful primary ulcer, at the site of inoculation (usually the external genital), and regional lymphadenitis

- It is a close differential of syphilis (where the ulcer is hard and painless), lymphogranuloma venerum, and herpes simplex infection
- *H. ducreyi* is best grown from scrapings of the ulcer base; on chocolate agar
- It requires X factor, but not V factor, for growth
- Treatment with **intramuscular ceftriaxone**, **oral co-trimoxazole** or **oral erythromycin** should heal the patient within 2 weeks

❖ BORDETELLA

- General characteristics of *Bordetella spp*
- They are small gram-ve bacilli
- They are obligate aerobes
- They are pathogenic in the human respiratory tract
- They produce toxins that causes skin necrosis

▪ Species
- The genus *Bordetella* has three pathogenic species: *B. pertussis, B. parapertussis, B. Bronchiseptica*

Specie	Disease	Growth on CM	Growth on B-G M	Oxidase test	Motility
B. pertussis	Pertussis	-	+	+	-
B. parapertussis	Parapertussis or classic pertussis (occasionally)	+	-	-	-
B. bronchiseptica	Chronic respiratory tract infection	+	-	+	+

CM is common media   B-GM is Bordet-Gengou medium

- Note that, of the three pathogenic species, only *B. pertussis* could not grow on common media, only *B. parapertussis* is oxidase-negative, and only *B. bronchiseptica* is motile

❖ **BORDETELLA PERTUSSIS**
- *B. pertussis* a.k.a. Bordet-Gengou bacilli, is the usually cause of pertussis (whooping cough)
- It is found only in the human respiratory tract; thus, is strictly a human pathogen

• **Peculiarities of *B. pertussis***
- It is a small, non-motile gram-ve bacilli
- Virulent strains are encapsulated with smooth colonies
- It is a nutritionally fastidious organism
- It is oxidase and catalase-positive
- It forms acid, but not gas, from glucose and lactose
- It produces hemolysis on blood-containing medium; X or V factor is not required for growth

▪ **Antigenic structures**

Antigenic structure	Characteristics and function
Filamentous hemagglutinin	Mediates adhesion to ciliated epithelial cells
Pertussis toxin	It is an exotoxin; the main virulence factor of *B. pertussis* Promotes lymphocytosis and sensitization to histamine It accounts for the paroxysmal cough typical of pertussis, and the prolonged immunity following infection
Tracheal cytotoxin	Inhibits DNA synthesis in ciliated epithelial cells; causing their death
Adenylate cyclase toxin	It is antiphagocytic
Lipopolysaccharide (endotoxin)	Destroys epithelial cells of the upper respiratory tract

- ▪ Mode of transmission
- – Through direct contact with respiratory secretions of infected patient or via droplets

- ▪ Pathogenesis
- – *B. pertussis* initially adhere to the ciliated epithelial cells of the nasopharynx, via the filamentous hemagglutinin and pili
- – They rapidly proliferate and spread onto the trachea and bronchi.
- – They elaborate the tracheal toxin, which interferes with ciliary action
- – The cessation of ciliary movement facilitates their entry into the epithelial cells
- – Within the cells, *B. pertussis* elaborates the pertussis toxin, which irritates the epithelial cells, causing the paroxysmal cough, and marked lymphocytosis
- – Invasion of underlying tissue or blood does not occur

- ▪ Clinical presentation
- – The clinical course of pertussis is divided into two stages:

- ● Catarrhal stage
- – This follows an incubation period of 2 weeks
- – During this period, patient is not very ill but is highly infectious
- – It is characterized by:
  - ● Mild coughing
  - ● Sneezing

- ● Paroxysmal stage
- – This stage is characterized by:
  - ● Paroxysmal cough (with the typical "whoop" upon inhalation)
  - ● Rapid exhaustion

- Vomiting
- Cyanosis
- Convulsions

- **Laboratory Diagnosis**
- ❖ Specimen: - saline nasal wash is preferred; nasopharyngeal swabs may as well be used

- **Culture**
- Media: - Bordet – Gengou medium or charcoal blood agar
- The small, non-motile, faintly staining gram-negative bacilli are identified by immunofluorescence staining
- Bordet – Gengou medium consist of potato, blood, and glycerol

- **Treatment**
- **Erythromycin** given during the catarrhal stage promotes elimination of the organisms
- Treatment after onset of paroxysmal phase rarely alters the clinical course.

- **Prevention**
Immunization

- Pertussis vaccine is usually administered in combination with toxoids of diphtheria and tetanus called Diphtheria-Pertussis-Tetanus (DPT) vaccine

- ❖ **BRUCELLA**
- This genus is named after David Bruce, an English physician, 1855-1931.

- **General characteristics of Brucella spp**
- They are aerobic gram-ve coccobacilli

- They are non-motile nonspore-forming, and non-encapsulated
- They live as facultative intracellular parasites
- They are primarily pathogenic in animals
- They cause brucellosis in animals, which may be transmitted to man; as zoonosis

- **Species of Brucella**
- There are a few different species of Brucella, each with slightly different host specificity:

Specie	Host
B. melitensis	Goat and sheep
B. abortus	Cattle
B. canis	Dogs
B. suis	Pigs
B. ovis	Sheep

- Note that, DNA studies have shown that only one specie exist in the genus, which is B. melitensis and others are biotypes

- **Transmission of Brucella**
- Direct contact with infected animals or their products
- Through ingestion of infected food or inhalation of aerosols
- Human to human transmission, for example through sexual intercourse or from mother to child, is exceedingly rare but possible.

- **Brucellosis**
- Brucellosis is a zoonotic diseases caused by *Brucella spp.*
- It causes infertility or abortion in affected animals
- In humans, it is a generalized infection characterized by:
    - Fever (which rises in the afternoon and fall at night, accompanied by drenching sweat)

- - Headache
- - Sweating
- - Malaise
- - Anorexia and weight loss
- - Lymphadenopathy and splenomegaly
- - Hepatitis and jaundice

- ▪ Diagnosis
- ❖ Specimen: - blood, bone marrow and lymph node biopsy for culture and serum for serology

- • Culture
- ❖ Media: - Castaneda medium
- – Brucella is isolated from a blood culture on Castaneda medium
- – Prolonged incubation period of up to 6weeks may be required; but with modern automated machines, positive result may be seen in 7days.
- – Brucella is differentiated from salmonella on blood culture using the urease test, which is positive for Brucella and negative for salmonella.

- • Serology
- – IgM and IgG antibodies to *Brucella* antigens can be detected in patient serum up to about 2 years after infection.
- – Though in *B. canis* infection, serologic tests may fail to detect antibodies

- ▪ Treatment
- – Combined treatment with a **tetracycline** (such as doxycycline) and either **streptomycin** for 2-3weeks or **rifampicin** for 6 weeks is the recommended treatment for human brucellosis

CHAPTER 14: MYCOBACTERIA

- Mycobacteria is a large genus of non-motile, non-spore-forming obligate aerobes
- Their uniqueness lies in their ability to resist decolorization by acid or alcohol once stained, thus, are also called acid-fast bacilli
- The genus is named after a long chain fatty acid present in their cell wall, called mycolic acid; which also accounts for their acid fastness

▪ Pathogenic Mycobacteria and their associated diseases

Mycobacteria	Disease
M. tuberculosis	Tuberculosis
M. bovis	Tuberculosis
M. leprae	Leprosy
M. ulcerans	Buruli ulcer
Mycobacterium avium complex	Tuberculosis-like disease, in immunocompromised patients
M. kansasii	Tuberculosis-like disease, in immunocompromised patients
M. scrofulaceum	Cervical lymphadenitis
M. chelonae and M. fortuitum	Skin infection and injection abscess

- Note that the triad of *M. tuberculosis, M. africanum,* and *M. bovis* is referred to as mycobacterium tuberculosis complex

• Growth characteristics of Mycobacteria
- All Mycobacteria except *M. leprae* grow aerobically on protein enriched media e.g. Lowenstein-Jensen medium
- Most species require increased CO_2 tension for growth
- Generally, saprophytic species grow faster, produce more pigment and are less acid fast, compared to the pathogenic species

- Classification of Mycobacteria

Classification criteria	Description	Example
Rate of growth		
Rapid growers	Grow in ≤ 7 days	*M. chelonae* and *M. fortuitum*
Slow growers	Grow in > 7 days	*M. tuberculosis, M. bovis, and M. ulcerans*
Pigment production		
Scotochromogens	Produces pigment when grown in both light and dark	*M. scrofulaceum*
Photochromogens	Produces pigment only in light	*M. kansasii*
Nonchromogens	Do not produce pigment	*M. tuberculosis* *M. ulcerans*

- *M. ulcerans* is the slowest growing mycobacterium
- *M. leprae* has never been cultivated in laboratory cell free culture media

❖ **MYCOBACTERIUM TUBERCULOSIS (Tuberculosis)**

- *M. tuberculosis* is a slow growing, nonchromogenic mycobacterium responsible for most cases of tuberculosis in humans
- Tuberculosis is a multisystemic chronic granulomatous disease characterised by chronic cough, hemoptysis, fever, and weight loss

- Virulence factors of *M. tuberculosis*

Virulence factor	Function
Cord factor	Inhibits leukocyte migration Causes chronic granulomas
Wax D	Induces the delayed type hypersensitivity reaction typical of tuberculosis
Sulfatides	Inhibit phagolysosome formation; ensuring

	intracellular survival of *M. tuberculosis*
Polysaccharides	Elicits immediate hypersensitivity reaction

- **Mode of transmission**
- Through inhalation of droplet nuclei released, when patient coughs, sneezes, or speaks

- **Risk factors**
- Overcrowding, undernutrition, immunosuppression, extremes of age, smoking, alcohol etc.

- **Pathogenesis**

- **Primary tuberculosis**
- Following inhalation, the bacilli reach the alveoli, and typically settle at the lower part of the upper lobe or the upper part of the lower lobe of the lung, just beneath the pleura
- Inflammatory response is triggered, and the bacilli are phagocytosed by alveolar macrophages, but they resist killing by preventing phagolysosome formation; thus, they create a primary lesion within the lungs called Ghon focus
- From the Ghon focus, organisms are carried to the hilar and mediastinal lymph nodes from where they may be disseminated to other body parts, via the hematogenous route
- Within the lymph nodes, inflammatory reaction against the bacilli creates an another lesion
- The combination of this lesion and the Ghon focus is called Ghon complex
- Since the macrophages could not destroy the bacilli, it presents them to the T-lymphocytes , causing a cell mediated immune response

- The sensitized T-cells in turn release interferon-γ and interleukin-2 which increase the bactericidal ability of the macrophages; hence most but not all the bacilli are destroyed
- The remaining bacilli remain dormant within the lungs, and when reactivated may cause secondary (post-primary) tuberculosis

• **Post-primary tuberculosis**

- This occurs in a previously sensitized host due to reactivation of the dormant bacilli (either spontaneously or due to immunosuppression) or less commonly, reinfection with new *M. tuberculosis*
- It is characterized by chronic tissue lesions, formation of tubercles, caseation, and fibrosis

▪ **Clinical features**

- Note that primary tuberculosis is asymptomatic in > 90% of patients

Symptoms	Signs
Pulmonary	**General**
Chronic cough	Wasting
Chest pain	Palor
Hemoptysis	Lymphadenopathy
Dyspnoea	Skin rash
	Finger clubbing
Constitutional	
Fever (low grade)	**Chest**
Weight loss	Consolidation
Anorexia	Pleura effusion
Night sweat	Lung collapse
Malaise	

- Laboratory diagnosis
- This is broadly divided into two:
  - Tuberculin skin test
  - Isolation and identification of *M. tuberculosis*

- Tuberculin skin test
- This is a test of skin reaction of an individual to a standard dose of tuberculoprotein
- It is a test of delayed hypersensitivity in a subject that has been infected by or immunized against *M. tuberculosis* at least 4-6 weeks ago
- There are three types: Mantoux test, Heaf test, and tine test; only Mantoux will be discussed:

- Mantoux test
- This is the most reliable of the three tests
- 0.1 ml of purified protein derivative (containing 5 tuberculin unit) is administered intradermally into the anterior forearm
- If an individual has been infected by or immunized against *M. tuberculosis* at least 4-6 weeks ago, an induration occurs at the site within 2-3 days

Result	Interpretation
Induration ≥ 10 mm	Positive for *M. tuberculosis* infection or immunization
Induration between 6-9 mm	Doubtful; may indicate infection by atypical Mycobacteria
Induration < 6 mm	Negative for *M. tuberculosis* infection
Induration > 15 mm	May indicate active *M. tuberculosis* infection

- Isolation and identification of *M. tuberculosis*
- These involve both microscopy and culture

❖ Specimen: - fresh sputum, gastric washings, urine, pleural fluid, CSF, joint fluid etc.

- Microscopy
- Basically, two types of staining technique are used for *M. tuberculosis* during microscopy:
- Non-fluorescence staining
- Fluorescence staining (see table 14.6)

Staining technique	Types	Result
Non-fluorescence staining	Ziehl-Neelsen (ZN) staining	AFB appear red on a blue background
	Kinyoun AFB staining	AFB appear red on a green background
Fluorescence staining	Auramine-rhodamine staining	AFB fluorescence orange-yellow

AFB- Acid-fast bacilli

- Culture
❖ Media: - Lowenstein-Jensen (LJ) medium, Middlebrook 7H10 medium, BACTEC etc.
- With LJ medium, *M. tuberculosis* growth is not detectable until after 4-6 weeks
- With BACTEC system, *M. tuberculosis* growth can be detected in 9-16 days

- Treatment
- First line drugs
- Mainly **isoniazid** and **rifampicin**; others are **pyrazinamide**, **ethambutol**, and **streptomycin**

- Second line drugs
- These drugs are more toxic, less effective, and more expensive; thus, they should be used only in cases of treatment failure or multi-drug resistance
- They are: kanamycin, capreomycin, ethionamide, cycloserine, ofloxacin, and ciprofloxacin.

CHAPTER 15: SPIROCHETES

- Spirochetes are long, slender, spiral or corkscrew shaped gram-negative bacteria, which though lack flagella, are capable of slow twisting motility

- Phylogeny
- The order Spirochaetales has two families: Spirochaetaceae (which are free-living) and Treponemataceae (which are human pathogens)
- The family Treponemataceae, which we are concerned, has three genera:
  - Genus *Treponema*
  - Genus *Borrelia*
  - Genus *Leptospira*

- Note that, the term "spirochete" applies to all microorganisms of the order Spirochaetales

- General characteristics of spirochetes
- They are long, slender, helically coiled, spiral-shaped gram-negative bacteria
- Within their periplasmic space are flagella-like organelles called endoflagella, with which they move

- ❖ GENUS TREPONEMA
- The genus *Treponema* comprise both pathogenic and non-pathogenic species, which are collectively referred to as treponemes

- Pathogenic treponemes and their associated diseases

Species	Disease
Treponema pallidum subspecies *pallidum*	Syphilis
Treponema pallidum subspecies	Yaws

pertenue	
Treponema pallidum subspecies *endemicum*	Endemic syphilis (bejel)
Treponema carateum	Pinta

❖ **TREPONEMA PALLIDUM SUBSPECIES PALLIDUM (SYPHILIS)**

- *T. pallidum* is the causative agent of syphilis; a sexually or congenitally transmissible multisystemic disease

▪ **Peculiarities of *T. pallidum***

- They are actively motile
- Dark field microscopy or immunofluorescent stain is required to observe them, as they are too thin to be seen on light microscopy
- They are stained by silver impregnation method, as they do not stain with aniline dyes e.g. crystal violet dye, safranin dye etc.
- They cannot be cultured on artificial media, chicks embryo or tissue culture
- They are rapidly killed by drying or elevated temperature

▪ **Forms of syphilis**

- Based on the mode of transmission of infection, syphilis can be divided to two forms:

• Acquired syphilis: - Syphilis transmitted through unprotected sexual intercourse with infected persons or through invasion of skin abrasion or intact mucosa by the organisms

• Congenital syphilis: - Syphilis transmitted through transplacental transfer of treponemes to the fetus

- Clinical course of syphilis
- Untreated syphilis usually progress through three clinical stages, with a latent phase in between the second and third stages; they are:
  - Primary syphilis
  - Secondary syphilis
  - ❖ Latent phase
  - Tertiary syphilis

- Primary syphilis
- Following entry, the treponemes multiply locally at the site; usually the genitals
- After an incubation period of 2-4 weeks, a papule develops at that site, which later breaks down to form a hard, painless, clean-based ulcer; called "hard chancre."
- The ulcer exudates serum containing numerous live treponemes, hence, is highly infectious
- The treponemes spread to regional lymph nodes, causing lymphadenopathy and bubo formation; and then to the blood stream
- After 2-8 weeks, the ulcer heals spontaneously, leaving only a small scar

- Secondary syphilis
- This follows the disappearance of chancre and blood stream invasion of the treponemes
- It is characterised chiefly by widespread mucocutaneous lesions over the entire body.
- The patient is highly infectious, as the lesions are rich in treponemes
- Other skin manifestations include painless, infectious genital lesions called condylomata lata, and patchy alopecia

- Systemic manifestations include malaise, fever, myalgias, arthralgias and lymphadenopathy
- Periosteitis, chorioretinitis, and aseptic meningitis may also accompany secondary syphilis

- **Latent phase**
- This is the stage at which all features of secondary syphilis have resolved, and thus, patient show no clinical sign of disease, but remain positive for serologic tests
- It is sub-divided into two phases: early latent phase and late latent phase
- Early latent phase, during which patient is prone to recurrence of the infectious skin lesions
- Late latent phase, during which patient is resistant to recurrence, but if pregnant, can transfer the infection to the unborn child
- About one-third of untreated patient go on to develop tertiary syphilis, whereas others remain asymptomatic for life

- **Tertiary syphilis**
- This stage is characterized by the development of granulomatous lesions in any organ of the body, but mainly the cardiovascular and central nervous system
- There are three categories of tertiary syphilis: cardiovascular syphilis, neurosyphilis, and gummatous syphilis

✓ **Cardiovascular syphilis**
- This manifests as aortitis, aortic aneurysm and aortic valve insufficiency

✓ **Neurosyphilis**
- This may manifests as meningovascular neurosyphilis and or parenchymatous neurosyphilis

- Meningovascular neurosyphilis is characterised by damage to the blood vessels of the meninges, brain and spinal cord.
- Parenchymatous neurosyphilis is characterised by destruction of neurons of the brain and spinal cord manifesting as generalised paralysis of the insane, tabes dorsalis, Argyll-Robertson pupil etc.

✓ **Gummatous syphilis**

- This is the development of granulomatous lesion, called gummas in any body organ, but mainly the liver, bones, and testes

✓ **Congenital syphilis**

- This is the form of syphilis resulting from transplacental transfer of treponemes to the fetus in an infected pregnant woman
- It may result in abortion or intra uterine fetal death, but more commonly, the child is born with various congenital defects, which include:
  - Widespread condylomata lata and rash
  - Rhinitis (snuffles)
  - Saddle nose (due to destruction of nasal septum)
  - Saber shins (due to inflammation and bowing of the tibia)
  - Hutchinson's teeth (widely spaced, notched upper incisors)
  - 8th cranial nerve deafness etc.

- Laboratory Diagnosis
❖ Specimen: - exudates for microscopy and serum for serology

• Microscopy
Dark field microscopy

- Typical twisting motility of live treponemes is seen in wet preparation of the syphilitic exudates

- **Fluorescent microscopy**
- Used to observe the typical fluorescence of antibody-bound treponemes after staining with fluorescein-labelled antitreponeme serum

- **Serology**
- This is the mainstay of diagnosis of syphilis
- They are divided into two: nontreponemal tests and treponemal antibody tests

✓ **Nontreponemal tests**
- These are used as screening tests for syphilis and for follow up of treatment
- They act by detecting specific antibodies to treponemes, IgM and IgG, in patient's serum using commercially prepared antigens such as cardiolipin-cholesterol-lecithin complex.
- They are not very sensitive in early syphilis, and false-positive results may occur
- Examples of nontreponemal tests include:
  - Venereal Disease Research Laboratory (VDRL)
  - Rapid plasma reagin (RPR) test

✓ **Treponemal antibody tests**
- These tests measure antibodies against *T. pallidum* antigens
- They are used to determine if a positive result from the nontreponemal test is truly positive
- Examples of treponemal antibody tests include:
  - *T. pallidum*-particle agglutination (TP-PA)
  - *T. pallidum* hemagglutination (TPHA)

- ▪ Treatment
- – **Penicillin** in concentration of 0.003Unit/mL/day is the treatment of choice for syphilis
- – Erythromycin, tetracyclines or ceftriaxone can be used in patients allergic to penicillin

- ▪ DISEASES RELATED TO SYPHILIS
- – These are diseases caused by treponemes closely related to *T. pallidum*
- – They all give positive treponemal and nontreponemal serologic tests for syphilis
- – However, none of them is sexually transmitted
- – All are commonly transmitted by direct contact
- – None of the causative organisms have been cultured on artificial media

- ❖ Treponema pallidum subspecies pertenue (Yaws)
- – *T. pertenue* is the causative agent of yaws; an endemic tropical disease affecting persons under age 15.
- – It is transmitted by direct contact with skin lesions or contaminated fomites

- ▪ Clinical manifestation
- – The primary lesion appears as a painless papule, which grows into a papilloma; called mother yaw
- – Mother yaw ulcerate, heals and leave a scar
- – This is followed by generalised secondary granulomatous papules that may relapse repeatedly
- – Late manifestations include destructive and deforming lesions of the skin bone and joints

- ▪ Laboratory diagnosis
- – Similar to those for syphilis

- Note that cross immunity may be between yaws and syphilis because, people with yaws do not develop syphilis

- Treatment
- penicillin (response is dramatic)

❖ Treponema carateum (Pinta)

- Pinta, caused by *T. carateum,* is an endemic tropical disease affecting all age groups
- It appears to be restricted to dark-skinned races, and is transmitted either by direct skin contact or flies.

- Clinical manifestation
- The primary lesion appears as a nonulcerating papule on exposed areas
- This is followed by appearance of flat hyperpigmented lesions on the skin
- Years afterwards, depigmentation and hyperkeratosis of the lesion occur
- Very rarely, the nervous and cardiovascular system may be involved

- Laboratory diagnosis
- Similar to those for syphilis
- No cross immunity occur between pinta and syphilis; thus, the patient can develop syphilis

- Treatment
- Penicillin

❖ GENUS BORELLIA

- Like the treponemes, members of the genus *Borrelia* belong to the order Spirochaetales and family Treponemataceae, and thus, are spirochetes

- Peculiarities of *Borrelia*
- They are larger and longer than the treponemes
- They are chiefly transmitted by arthropods e.g. tick and louse
- They can be stained by ordinary dyes such as Gram stains; with which they are gram-negative

- Species

Species	Vector	Disease
Borrelia recurrentis	Body louse	Louse-borne relapsing fever
Borrelia hermsii, Borrelia duttonii etc.	Tick of the genus *Ornithodoros*	Tick-borne relapsing fever
Borrelia burgdorferi	Ticks of the genus *Ixodes*	Lyme disease

❖ **BORRELIA RECURRENTIS AND BORRELIA HERMSII (Relapsing Fever)**
- Relapsing fever is an acute, systemic, usually self-limited disease, characterised by alternating periods of febrile and afebrile episodes, with spirochetemia during the febrile episodes but not during the intervals
- Based on the causative organism, there are two main forms of relapsing fever:
  - Louse-borne relapsing fever (epidemic form) - *Borrelia recurrentis*
  - Tick-borne relapsing fever (endemic form) - *Borrelia hermsii, Borrelia duttonii* etc.

117

- Pathophysiology of relapsing fever
- Incubation period is 3-10days
- The spirochetes multiply at the portal of entry, and enter the blood; causing spirochetemia and sudden onset of high grade fever and chills
- Fever subsides after 3-5 days, due to their clearance from the blood, leaving the patient weak but not ill.
- After an afebrile episode of 4-10days, a second attack of fever, chills, intense headache and malaise occur
- These may re-occur for about 3 to 10 times, however with decreasing severity due to development of antibodies against the spirochetes by the host

- Laboratory diagnosis
- Specimen: - blood taken during the rise of fever, for microscopy and animal inoculation

- Microscopy
- Thin or thick blood smears shows coiled spirochetes among the red cells

- Animal inoculation
- White mice are inoculated intraperitoneally with blood.
- Stained films of tail blood are examined for spirochetes after 2-4 days

- Treatment
- Penicillin, tetracyclines and erythromycin are effective

- ❖ BORRELIA BURGDORFERI (Lyme disease)
- Lyme disease is a recurrent, multisystemic disorder characterised by migratory skin lesion called erythema

migrans, along with flu-like symptoms and late manifestation of arthralgia and arthritis; caused by *B. burgdorferi*
- Lyme disease is named after a town called Lyme in Connecticut, where it occurred in epidemics among children
- It is transmitted by bite of ticks of the genus *Ixodes*

- **Pathophysiology**
- After injection of *B. burgdorferi,* by the tick, the organisms migrate out of the site, producing the characteristic skin lesion, erythema migrans.
- The organisms is then disseminated via lymphatics or blood to other skin, musculoskeletal sites and many body organs
- The antibodies produced against the organism is anti-flagellar, and thus non-protective
- The antibodies however form complexes with antigens, and are deposited in the skin, joints and other tissues
- This initiate a type III hypersensitivity reaction leading to tissue destruction

- **Clinical features**

Stage	Feature
1 (days-weeks)	Erythema migrans, fever, chills, myalgias, and headache
2 (weeks-months)	Arthralgia, arthritis, meningitis, facial nerve palsy, radiculopathy
3 (months-years)	Chronic skin, nervous system, and joint involvement

- **Laboratory diagnosis**
- Specimen: - blood for serology, CSF or joint fluid can also be used.

- Serology
- This is the mainstay of diagnosis of Lyme disease
- It is based on the detection of the antibodies against *B. burgdorferi* in the serum of a symptomatic patient

- Microscopy
- *B. burgdorferi* can been found in sections of biopsy specimens
- However, examination of stained specimen is not a sensitive method for diagnosis

- Treatment
- Doxycycline or amoxicillin is effective

CHAPTER 16: CHLAMYDIA

- The genus chlamydia is unique because its members are obligate intracellular parasites i.e. they cannot survive outside their host cell
- They lack the mechanisms required for the synthesis of metabolic energy; thus are restricted to an intracellular existence, where the host cell supplies energy-rich intermediates

- Peculiarities of the genus chlamydia
- They are regarded as gram-negative, as their cell wall retain the red of safranin dye
- Their cell wall lack muramic acid
- They are sensitive to inhibitors of cell wall synthesis (e.g. penicillin)
- They all exhibit similar morphologic features and share a common group antigen

- Species
- Three species of the genus chlamydia are pathogenic to man:
  - *Chlamydia trachomatis*
  - *Chlamydia pneumoniae*
  - *Chlamydia psittaci*

- Developmental cycle of chlamydiae
- Chlamydiae exist in two forms during development:
- Elementary body
- Reticulate (initial) body

- Elementary body
- A metabolically inert, small infectious particle
- Has an electron dense nucleoid

- Reticulate body
- Formed when the elementary body enters a host cell
- It is large and devoid of electron dense nucleoid
- It grows in size and divides repeatedly by binary fission to form new elementary bodies
- The host cell rupture to release the elementary bodies, which in turn infect other cells

❖ **CHLAMYDIA TRACHOMATIS**
- Humans are the natural hosts of *C. trachomatis*, in whom it causes infections of the eye, genitals, and respiratory tract

▪ Trachoma
- A chronic keratoconjunctivitis (inflammation of the conjunctiva and cornea) characterised by photophobia, pain, and lacrimation
- It may progress to corneal scarring and blindness, but systemic symptoms are rare

- Genital tract infection and inclusion conjunctivitis
- In male: *C. trachomatis* causes non-gonococcal urethritis and occasionally epididymitis
- In female: it causes non-gonococcal urethritis, cervicitis, and pelvic inflammatory disease, which may lead to sterility or ectopic pregnancy
- Inclusion conjunctivitis resembles trachoma closely, it occurs when genital secretions of infected adult is self-inoculated onto the conjunctiva
- Newborn acquire the infection during passage through an infected birth canal

- Neonatal pneumonia
- Newborns of infected mother may develop pneumonia within 2-12 weeks of birth

- Lymphogranuloma venerum
- A sexually transmitted disease caused by *C. trachomatis*
- It starts as a painless papule on the genitals, which heals spontaneously
- The bacteria migrate to regional lymph node causing its enlargement for about 2 months
- The node becomes increasingly tender and may break open to release purulent secretions

❖ CHLAMYDIA PNEUMONIAE
- Human are the only known host of *C. pneumoniae*
- It causes atypical pneumonia in young adults world wide
- It usually involve both upper and lower respiratory tract
- Most infections are usually mild or asymptomatic

❖ CHLAMYDIA PSITTACI
- Birds are the natural host of *C. psittaci*
- Humans are infected by inhaling *C. psittaci* laden dust from poultry product
- It infects the lungs primarily; producing severe pneumonia and sepsis
- It is associated with high mortality rate; though, infection may be mild in some cases

▪ Laboratory diagnosis
- Culture
- Chlamydiae are isolated using tissue culture cells, embryonated eggs or mice

- Serology
- This is based on detection of chlamydia antigen in exudates or urine, by ELISA

- **Treatment**
  - Tetracycline e.g. doxycycline
  - Macrolides e.g. erythromycin, clarithromycin, azithromycin

CHAPTER 17: RICKETTSIA

- Like chlamydia, *rickettsia* are obligate intracellular parasite, as they are unable to produce sufficient energy to replicate extracellularly
- They are small gram-negative coccobacilli, and except for Q fever (*Coxiella burnetii*), are transmitted to human by arthropods, via the skin

- Properties of *Rickettsia*
- They are readily visible under the light microscope, when appropriately stained
- They grow readily in yolk sac of embryonated egg, cell culture and experimental animals
- Their cell wall include muramic acid and diaminopimelic acid (being gram-negative)
- Their growth is enhanced by sulphonamides (co-trimoxazole) thus should be avoided in treating their infection
- Tetracyclines and chloramphenicol, can be therapeutically effective
- They divide by binary fission within the host cells

- Species
- Based on the specific disease they cause, species under the genus *Rickettsia* are grouped into three

Spotted fever group	Typhus group	Scrub Typhus group	Q fever
Rickettsia rickettsii *Rickettsia akari* *Rickettsia australis* *Rickettsia conorii*	*Rickettsia prowazekii* *Rickettsia typhi*	*Orientia tsutsugamushi*	*Coxiella burnetii*

- **DISEASES CAUSED BY *RICKETTSIA***

- Rocky Mountain spotted fever
  - Caused by *Rickettsia rickettsii*
  - Transmitted by bite of an infected tick
  - It resembles typhus clinically, however the pattern of rash does not correlate
  - Fatality is up to 50% in untreated elderly cases, but lower for young adults and children

✓ **Clinical features**
  - Sudden onset of fever and chills
  - Petechial rash that appears early and spreads from the limbs upwards onto the trunk and face
  - Myalgias
  - Severe headache
  - Prostration

- Q fever
  - This is an acute, generally self-limited infection caused by *Coxiella burnetii*
  - Transmitted by air borne fomites (very rarely by tick)
  - Rash is not a feature of this disease
  - Blood culture is usually negative but there is increased antibody titre to *C. burnetii*

✓ **Clinical features**
  - Fever and chills, malaise, myalgia, and headache
  - May be complicated by mild pneumonia, hepatitis and endocarditis

- Epidemic typhus (louse-borne typhus)
  - Caused by *Rickettsia prowazekii*
  - Transmitted by bite of an infected louse

- Human are the major reservoir of this organisms
- It is characterised by abrupt onset of chills, fever, and malaise; headache of increasing severity, backache, myalgia and skin rash
- CNS symptoms include dullness to stupor and at times coma and death

- **Endemic typhus (flea-borne typhus)**
- Caused by *Rickettsia typhi*
- Transmitted by bite of an infected flea
- Clinical feature are milder forms of that of epidemic typhus; thus fatality rarely occurs except in the elderly

- **Scrub typhus (mite-borne typhus)**
- This is an acute infectious disease that resembles epidemic typhus clinically
- Caused by *Orientia tsutsugamushi*
- Transmitted by bite of an infected mite larvae
- It is characterized by a pathognomonic primary cutaneous lesion or eschar at the site of inoculation
- Other features are regional lymphadenopathy, fever, head ache and rash

- **Laboratory diagnosis**

- **Serology**
- The most widely used serological tests are indirect fluorescent antibody technique which detects IgM and IgG specific for the *Rickettsia* antigen

- **Culture**
- Isolation of *Rickettsia* is technically difficult and is of limited usefulness in diagnosis

- It requires viable eukaryotic cells, such as antibiotic free cell culture, embryonated eggs and susceptible animals

■ Treatment

- **Tetracyclines** and **chloramphenicol** are effective

CHAPTER 18: MYCOPLASMA

- *Mycoplasma is a* genus of small cell wall-free bacteria under the family Mycoplasmataceae
- They are unique in microbiology because of their extremely small size and their ability to grow and replicate on laboratory media

- Peculiarities of *Mycoplasma*
- They lack cell wall, but are bound by a flexible triple-layered cell membrane
- They are completely resistant to inhibitors of cell wall synthesis e.g. penicillins and cephalosporins
- They are sensitive to inhibitors of protein synthesis such as tetracycline and erythromycin
- They can replicate independent of their host, and can grow on complex but cell-free media unlike *Chlamydiae* and *Rickettsia.*
- Their colony frequently have a characteristic fried egg shape; with a raised centre and thinner outer edges
- They are the only bacteria that have cholesterol (a sterol of the eukaryotic cell membrane) on their membrane

- Species
- There are over 150 species in the genus *Mycoplasma*; however, about 17 of them are of human origin, only four of which are of medical importance; they include:
  - *Mycoplasma pneumoniae*
  - *Mycoplasma hominis*
  - *Ureaplasma urealyticum*
  - *Ureaplasma parvum*

- Mycoplasma pneumoniae
- *M. pneumoniae* is a prominent cause of atypical pneumonia, especially in individuals between 5-20 years

- They are termed "atypical" because the clinical presentation of their pneumonia deviates from the classical pattern seen with other etiologic organisms
- It is transmitted from person to person by means of infected respiratory secretions
- Clinical spectrum ranges from asymptomatic to serious pneumonitis; however, the disease is usually mild

- **Clinical features**
- Malaise
- Fever (low-grade)
- Headache
- Chills (no rigor)
- Sore throat (scratchy)
- Persistent, slowly worsening cough; initially non-productive, but later may produced blood-streaked sputum

- **Laboratory diagnosis**

- **Microscopy**
- Sputum Gram stain is done to rule out other bacterial pathogens e.g. *S. pneumoniae*

- **Serology**
- Using compliment fixation tests, there is a rise in specific antibodies to *M. pneumoniae* by 4-folds between the acute and convalescent phase sera
- Enzyme immunoassay (EIA) may be done to detect IgM and IgG antibodies; it is highly sensitive and specific, but may not be readily available

- **Polymerase chain reaction**
- PCR assay of specimens may also be done; but is not routine investigation

- **Treatment**
  - **Tetracyclines** and **erythromycins** can produce clinical improvement but do not eradicate the mycoplasmas

Thank you for reading! If you enjoyed this book or found it useful

I would be very grateful if you would post a short review on Amazon.

Your support really does make a difference and I read all the reviews personally so I can get your feedback and make this book even better.

Thank you.

Printed in Great Britain
by Amazon

29507179R00076